Concussion, Traumatic Brain Injury, mTBI
The ultimate TBI rehabilitation guide

Concussion, Traumatic Brain Injury, mTBI The ultimate TBI rehabilitation guide

Your holistic manual for traumatic brain injury rehabilitation and care

Leon Edward and Dr Anum Khan

Table of Contents

Introduction

It normally starts with pain, and then darkness, deep darkness. And when you "wake up" you are not really awake at all. Your new awareness is often a dull sense of confusion. When you finally come back to the world and your senses once again serve you rather than deceive you, everything is different, especially you.

Who are these people? What are they doing to me now? Why am I hurting so much? These questions are slowly answered as you regain clarity. And when the emergency care and operations and medicines and machines and surgeons and nurses and equipment and prodding and heroic intervention stop, you start on a new road, a road less travelled, a road to become the new you, a completely new version of yourself that you have to go out and look for, that you have to become and embrace.

This is a difficult journey for most of us, not to mention loved ones and family, because as you suffer, so they suffer, and as you change, so they change, and as you battle, so they bleed too.

The good news that I want to share with everyone that face this disruptive and undoubtedly traumatic journey, to paraphrase Mark Twain, is *that reports of my hopelessness are greatly exaggerated*[i] .

You can – survive, and more – you can become you again. Maybe a slightly changed you, but everyone changes over time, not so? In this book, I attempt to add to the available information out there by sharing what I needed and wanted to know during my own dark days. There are vast amounts of data & information available on the web, and in this work, I attempted to sort and organize some of it to be ready, and at hand when it is needed quickly.

CHAPTER 1

Understanding the Mechanics

TRAUMATIC BRAIN INJURIES

Traumatic brain injury (TBI) occurs when a blow to the head causes brain damage. TBI includes anything from mild concussions up to severe brain damage. Treatment can range from rest only to intensive care and emergency surgery. Survivors can face a lifetime of disruptions, physical and mental impairment severe cognitive changes. Most patients will undergo long-term rehabilitation, and some might even need to relearn basic skills.

MAIN CAUSES OF TRAUMATIC BRAIN INJURIES

In the United States, the most common causes of TBI include falls (35.2%), motorcycle and car accidents, automobile accidents involving pedestrians (17.3%) and assaults (10%) with or without a weapon. Athletics and sports also cause a lot of TBI. In the U.S., combat head injuries are also pervasive. Combat injuries combine blunt (closed head injuries), penetrating (with retained fragments, perforating, grooving the skull, tangential and cranial facial degloving) and blast-over pressure CNS injuries. Approximately one and a half million people suffer TBI annually in the United States. Fifty-two thousand people die, and 1.365 million people are treated and released, while another 275,000 people are hospitalized with moderate to severe symptoms. More than 30,000 children have disabled annually. The estimated cost of TBI annually exceeds $48 billion.

PRIMARY AND SECONDARY TRAUMATIC BRAIN INJURIES

The primary injury, caused at the moment of impact, can involve a specific part of the brain, or it can affect the entire brain. The skull does not have to be fractured. The impact of the blow to the head might cause the brain to literally crash against the inside of the skull repeatedly as it moves back and forth. The impact can cause bruising, bleeding and tearing of nerve fibers.

Directly after the impact, symptoms might be absent. Often though, the condition of the patient can deteriorate very rapidly. At first, the patient might be confused. Memory and vision might be impaired, and dizziness and even unconsciousness might follow.

The brain often experiences delayed trauma. Swelling, when it occurs, can push the brain against the skull, and this might reduce the flow of blood and access to oxygen. Injuries resulting from trauma are classified as secondary injuries. The secondary injuries are very often more detrimental than the primary injuries were.

TBI ARE CLASSIFIED INTO THREE MAIN CATEGORIES, DEPENDING ON SEVERITY

Mild TBI (Concussions included) will, if at all, result in only brief loss of consciousness, and the patient will normally be awake – with eyes open. Symptoms might include a headache, disorientation, confusion, and loss of memory.

Moderate TBI will lead to loss of consciousness between twenty minutes and six hours. The patient will be sluggish and inert, but the eyes will open to stimulation. A degree of brain swelling or bleeding will present, and this will lead to sleepiness. But, the patient will be able to wake up when prompted.

Severe TBI leads to unconsciousness for longer than six hours. The eyes will respond to any stimulation and will not open.

BRAIN ANATOMY

The central nervous system dictates our thoughts and feelings and our movement and activities with the information received from our nerve cells, mind and environment. The main parts of our central nervous system are the brain, the spinal cord and the nerves throughout the body.

The brain is divided into two halves. The two halves (hemispheres) work together to command our thoughts and behaviors. The left hemisphere controls movements of the right side of the body. It also controls reasoning, speaking, writing and numerical skills. The right side controls the left side of the body's movements and is the center of insight and imagination, awareness of the multi-dimensional nature of reality (three dimensions), creativity and musical ability as well as our interpretation skills.

Each hemisphere of the brain is further divided into smaller parts or lobes. The frontal lobe is responsible for the most important movements of the eyes, the trunk, and the extremities. This is where memory is located, judgment as well as the control mechanisms to moderate behavior.

Behind the frontal lobe, the parietal lobe controls the remaining movements and the senses, as well as our perception and sense of space. Alongside the frontal and parietal lobes, we find the temporal lobe. The temporal lobes are co-responsible for memory, controls language and are crucial in the experience and control of emotions.

At the back of the brain, we find the occipital lobe, which interprets what we see with our eyes. These lobes are all part of the cerebrum of the brain.

Under the cerebrum, just above the brainstem, the cerebellum controls our coordination and timing. The brainstem – also popularly known as the reptile brain – is responsible for the automatic functions in the body. This includes breathing, blood pressure and arousal. The slightest injury to the brainstem can lead to coma or a very low level of consciousness.

Table 1.1	HEALTHY BRAIN	INJURED BRAIN
BRAINSTEM	Controls all the automatic functions in the body – breathing, digestion, heart rate, temperature	Vertigo, dizziness, Impaired balance and difficulty of movement, difficulty in swallowing, changes in breathing
CEREBELLUM	Balance timing. Coordination.	Slurred speech. Dizziness. Tremors. Loss of dexterity. Difficulty walking.
FRONTAL LOBE	Movement, memory, concentration, intelligence, behavior control, judgment.	Changes in behavior and emotional life. Impaired language skills. Impaired judgment. Memory loss. Loss of motivation. Loss of inhibition. Impaired mental capacity. Paralysis (left or right side of the body)
OCCIPITAL LOBE	Visual interpretation	Visual impairment. Illusions & Hallucinations. Impaired ability to read and write.
PARIETAL LOBE	Reading & writing & vocabulary. Movement. Sensation. Spatial perception	Impaired reading, writing, and vocabulary. Impaired hand-eye coordination and loss of mathematical reasoning.
TEMPORAL LOBE	Emotional regulation, memory and language.	Memory loss. Changes in sexuality. Aggression. Facial recognition problems. Seizures. Loss of the ability to understand language.

TYPES OF INJURY

It is easy enough in theory, to distinguish and classify the different types of brain injury. In real time, traumatic brain injuries rarely exist in isolation. More often than not, the patient will suffer a combination of injuries that overlap, each presenting a different level of severity. When more than one region of the brain is injured, it is rarely possible to pinpoint the specific location of injury in isolation.

Primary injuries can be further broken down into closed head injuries, caused by the external impact that does not fracture the skull, and open head injury, where the skull is penetrated (fractured) and skull fragments or foreign objects (i.e., bullets) are pushed into the brain.

PRIMARY INJURIES

Concussion

A concussion is a mild injury to the head that can cause a brief loss of consciousness but does not normally bring about permanent brain injury. A concussion is a diffuse injury, which means it is spread over a large area and cannot be pinpointed to a specific location. Normally a concussion will present as an overall decrease in levels of consciousness.

Contusion

When an impact to the head leaves a bruise to a specific area of the brain. This is also known as *coup or counter-coup* injuries. In *coup* injuries, the brain is injured directly under the point of impact while in *countercoup* injuries the brain it is injured on the opposite side of the impact. Contusions are focal injuries – that is to say, the injury is not spread out (diffuse), but it is specific to a location. Focal injuries will have symptoms based on the region of the brain injured, as seen in table 1.1 above.

Diffuse Axonal Injury

Axons, which compose what is also known as the white matter of the brain, connect nerve cells throughout the brain. When the brain reverberates (quickly moves back and forth inside the skull), the nerve axons are torn and damaged. During automobile accidents, for example, rapid rotation or deceleration of the brain causes stretching of these nerve cells on a cellular level, the brain's normal transmission of signals (information) is disrupted, and this can dramatically impact the person's alertness and wakefulness.

Ischemia is another form of diffuse injury. This happens when certain parts of the brain are cut off from an adequate supply of blood. A marked decrease in blood supply is especially perilous for a TBI patient because the brain becomes extremely sensitive even the smallest decreases in blood supply after a traumatic injury. Changes in blood pressure during the first-week post- head injury can have adverse effects.

Hematoma

When a blood vessel in the brain is ruptured, bleeding starts and the blood naturally clots. Sometimes these hematomas are very small. When a hematoma is large, it might compress the brain. Symptoms will depend on the location of the hematoma and hematomas are named for their location. A hematoma that forms between the skull and the dura (the tough outermost membrane enveloping the brain and spinal cord) is named an epidural hematoma. When the hematoma forms between the brain and the dura, it is named a subdural hematoma. When the hematoma forms deep inside the brain, it is named an intracerebral hematoma. Under fortunate circumstances, the body will reabsorb the hematoma. Large clots (hematomas) are periodically removed by surgery.

Second Impact Syndrome (SIS)

SIS causes the brain to swell catastrophically. SIS is not strictly speaking a type of injury, rather an extreme response of the brain to a second blow to the head/brain (even a very mild blow) after a first impact (seconds up to days after the first blow) already changed the brains functioning and left it in a vulnerable state. A second blow to the head during concussion unleashes a series of metabolic events that might start within 15 seconds. One of the ramifications is a very large increase in blood flow due to a loss of autoregulation of the brain's blood vessels. Huge increases in intracranial pressure follow, and this might cause cerebellar herniation (the brain is squeezed past structures within the skull) which is very often fatal.

Skull Fracture

Linear skull fractures are simple cracks or breaks in the skull. The bigger concern when this happens is the fear that the underlying force that created the fracture might have caused damage to the brain itself. Fractures to the base of the skull can be very problematic because it may cause damage to arteries, nerves and other structures. If a fracture reaches down to the sinuses, this may cause cerebrospinal fluid to leak from the nose and ears. Sometimes this might require intervention to insert a lumbar drain. Depressed skull fractures are more problematic. These fractures happen when a part of the bone presses on or into the brain itself. This more often than not requires surgical intervention. The specific damage caused will be dependent upon the region where this fracture happens as well as its interaction/coexistence with any diffuse brain injuries.

Traumatic Subarachnoid Hemorrhage

When an escape of blood from a ruptured blood vessel leaks into the space that surrounds the brain, this kind of stroke caused by an external impact on the brain, is described as a subarachnoid hemorrhage. The subarachnoid space is the fluid-filled space around the brain between the arachnoid membrane and the pia mater (the delicate innermost membrane enveloping the brain and spinal cord) through which major blood vessels pass. The cerebrospinal fluid in this space forms a floating cushion the brain hovers in for protection. When an injury causes some of the small arteries to tear, the blood flow spreads all over the surface of the brain, causing widespread traumatic effects.

TABLE 1.2   SECONDARY INJURIES

SYMPTOMS OF SECONDARY BRAIN INJURY
Amnesia
Attention deficit
Bewilderment
Convulsions
Depression
Disorganization
Disrupted sleep
Emotionality
Exhaustion
Headaches
Impaired vision
Loss of Consciousness
Moodiness
Nausea & Vomiting
Unsteadiness
Vertigo

Edema

After the initial injury to the brain, swelling can occur for up to five days. The swelling often happens gradually because of the body's reaction to the primary injury. In order to heal the initial injury, the body accumulates extra fluid and nutrients to the site of the injury to attempt to heal itself. Such inflammation in the brain can be quite dangerous. The skull is rigid, and space for extra fluid and nutrients is limited. As the brain swells, the pressure inside the skull is increased, and this can result in brain cell damage as well as blood flow interruption (ischemia).

TABLE 1.3   POSSIBLE OUTCOMES OF TBI

PHYSICAL PROBLEMS	COGNITIVE PROBLEMS	BEHAVIORAL PROBLEMS
Coordination problems	Attention deficit	Inappropriate behavior
Paralysis	Confusion	Lack of self-awareness
Sexual impairment	Impaired language skills	Loss of empathy
Speech impairment	Loss of abstract understanding	Irritability
Tiredness	Loss of reading & writing skills	Anger
Vertigo	Impaired learning skills	Lack of emotional control
Weakness	Impaired problem solving	Depression.
	Lack of judgment	Mood swings
	Impaired memory	Loss of drive
		Dependency
		Restlessness
		Frustration
		Selfishness
		Sluggishness

PREVENTION OF TRAUMATIC BRAIN INJURIES

Prevention is better than cure. This still holds true, especially for traumatic brain injuries which are to a very large degree preventable.

Headgear & Protection

Millions of people can be protected from traumatic brain injuries by simply wearing protective gear when participating in certain activities. By selecting the best headgear available, safety can be maximized. Whether riding a bicycle, skateboard, motorcycling or driving an all-terrain vehicle, wearing the required safety and head gear will improve your chances considerably. This is especially true when participating in sports. Football, hockey, and numerous other sports require headgear. Choosing and fitting the right headgear that fits well, is essential. When driving, always wear a seatbelt. Make sure that all children are secured and that age-appropriate child safety seats are properly secured to the car and to the child.

Alcohol & Drugs

One of the leading causes of vehicular accidents and accidents involving pedestrians is intoxication. Driving – or even walking – while under the influence of drugs and alcohol is dangerous. No one should ever get behind the wheel of a car or walk where there is any traffic, while even slightly intoxicated. The same goes for diabetics who use insulin and patients on medication. Do not drive when you are vulnerable to either the side effects of medication or the condition the medication is used for. People with poor eyesight must have their eyes checked regularly, and those with night-blindness must stay off the roads after dusk. Sensitive eyes can be protected and enhanced by wearing suitable sunglasses.

Exercise and Fitness

Falls account for a very large proportion of all traumatic brain injuries. One of the primary preventative strategies to prevent falls are exercises that can enhance dexterity, coordination, and balance, and improve strength and stamina. This is especially true for the elderly. Falls more often than not, occurs in the home. Decluttering the home by removing items from the floor and installing safety equipment (non-slip mats in the bathtub; handrails on stairways) can improve safety by a large margin. Adequate lighting on stairways can make a difference. By placing bars on the windows, children can be prevented from falling.

Firearms, Weapons and High Crime Areas

It is advisable to store firearms in a safe or locked cabinet and to store the ammunition separately. When entering a high crime zone, vigilance improves safety. Crowded spaces known for low levels of control, like bars and some restaurants and clubs, can be dangerous too. Again, avoiding these zones altogether or remaining very vigilant, can help prevent possible injury.

DIAGNOSIS OF TRAUMATIC BRAIN INJURIES

When a patient arrives at the emergency room with head injuries, time is of the essence. Doctors need to assess the patient's condition very quickly to determine the damage. This is done by finding out as much as possible about how the injury happened and what the patient's symptoms are.

GLASGOW COMA SCORE (GCS)

The Glasgow Coma Score (GCS) is the industry standard. The GCS is a fast 15-point test to grade the patient's level of consciousness in order to determine whether the injury is mild, moderate or severe. The patient is asked to *open his/her eyes,* to respond to orientation questions like *name, or date,* and to follow commands like *hold up two fingers or show a thumbs-up.* If the patient is unconscious or unable to follow commands, his/her response to painful stimuli is checked. Each response is graded according to the GCS scorecard and added together. Scores range from three to fifteen, a score of 13 – 15 indicates mild TBI; a score of 9-12 indicates a moderate TBI and a score of eight and below, indicates severe traumatic brain injury.

DIAGNOSTIC IMAGING TESTS

Computed Tomography (CT)

A CT scan takes X-ray images from different angles around the head and by using advanced computer algorithms then create cross-sectional images stacked over each other of the bones, blood vessels and soft tissue inside the head and the brain. In this way, detailed images of the anatomical structures of the brain become visible. A scan of the head taken as soon after the injury as possible can help to identify the extent of the damage and the presence of hematomas, bleeding, and fractures. CT scans remain useful throughout the treatment and recovery phase to monitor the evolution of the injury and to aid in making decisions about treatment.

Magnetic Resonance Imaging (MRI)

MRI scans are especially useful for examining the soft tissues of the brain and spinal cord. An MRI uses a large magnet combined with radio waves to give a detailed view of organs and structures inside the body. This is very helpful for the diagnoses of various conditions. Sometimes a contrast agent (dye) might be injected into the patient's bloodstream. An MRI scan complements the CT scan – it can detect subtle changes in the brain that is invisible to the CT scan.

Magnetic Resonance Spectroscopy(MRS)

The MRS scan uses a large magnet combined with radiofrequency waves to feed signals to a computer that creates detailed images. These tests are added to the MRI scan of the brain after the MRS analyzes molecules like hydrogen ions and protons to measure the chemical metabolism of the brain. The numerical analysis generated this way provides prognoses for the patient's ability to recover from injury.

ACUTE MANAGEMENT AND TREATMENT OPTIONS

Neurosurgery

If there is a hematoma (clot) large enough to damage the brain, a cerebral edema, or a pooling of blood, surgery will be required. A flap of bone is removed from the skull over the site of the clot. The clot is removed, and the arteries will be repaired. The skull heals rapidly, and the operation is usually straightforward and without much risk.

If the skull was penetrated and the wound goes through to the brain, surgery will also take place. With proper treatment, these wounds normally heal very well. A future tendency to develop epileptic seizures (post-traumatic epilepsy) can occur. This can be treated with medication to reduce the risk.

Neurosurgery is very time-consuming, and recovery can take a long time because of the injury to the brain. The severity of the brain injury, rather than the skill of the surgeon, is often the main determinant of success.

Intensive Care

After surgery, the patient will be moved to the intensive care unit (ICU) where treatment and condition will be monitored 24-hours per day. Heart rate, blood pressure, brain function, food, and fluid intake will be monitored continually.

Intracranial pressure will be monitored by the insertion of an intracranial pressure monitor (ICP).

A brain oxygen monitor (Licox) is placed through a small hole in the skull and positioned in the brain tissue. The oxygen levels and the temperature of the brain are constantly monitored. Oxygen is optimized for the brain to heal.

A cerebral blood flow monitor (Hemedex) is placed next to the Licox to evaluate blood flow throughout the brain.

For some patients, a ventilator might be needed to help them to breathe. It is connected to the patient via an endotracheal tube placed into the patient's mouth and down the windpipe. The machine can then push air in and out of the lungs.

A feeding tube will be added to patients on a ventilator and with decreased alertness. A nasal gastric feeding tube may be inserted and passed down the throat to the stomach for delivery of liquid nutrition and medication delivery.

To monitor the patient for seizures due to abnormal electrical discharge from the brain, all TBI patients will be monitored with an EEG (electroencephalogram) for 72 hours after the injury.

Medication

Medication will form a critical part of the acute management phase of treatment. Pain medication is normally offered for all patients who have more injuries than just head wounds. It is often necessary to sedate patients with severe traumatic brain injuries. These sedatives can be quickly turned off to awaken the patient and check for alertness and mental status.

To control the intracranial pressure of the brain hypertonic saline is used to draw out extra water from the brain cells and to drain it through the blood vessels to the kidneys where it can be filtered out of the blood.

Because patients with moderate to severe brain injuries are prone to seizure during the first week after the injury, patients are given anti-seizure medications to prevent the same.

Infections are always are a risk, irrespective of all the preventative measures taken. Any device placed within the patient can introduce a microbe into the system. If an infection is suspected, tests will be done, and if so, antibiotics will be introduced as treatment.

Recovery

Every head injury is unique, and patients recover at different rates and varying degrees. No one knows when a patient will comprehend and interact with caregivers. Recovery can take weeks, months and years. The recovery process normally goes through stages: coma, confusion, amnesia, recovery.

Coma

The brain waves of a person in a coma are very different from the waves of a sleeping person. Movements of the eyes during a coma are just basic reflexes or automatic responses to stimuli.

When the patient starts to wake up, self-protection is turned on, and the patient will often move away from any stimuli and tend to try and remove any attachments that irritate them. The patient is most likely not aware of his surroundings yet and may respond in the same way to all stimuli. Signs might be an increased breathing rate, moaning, moving and sweating, as well as an increased blood pressure level.

When the patient starts to wake up, their interactions will become more purposeful. They might look at and follow visitors with their eyes or respond to simple commands. Confusion, inappropriate and agitated behavior are very likely.

MILD TBI (CONCUSSION)

Mild TBI (MTBI) is another name for a concussion. MTBI can happen without the patient's awareness. No loss of consciousness has to occur, and no physical signs of a head injury have to be present. Normally MTBI does not lead to any significant brain injury.

MTBI is caused by rapid acceleration or deceleration of the brain after a bump, blow or jolt to the head, or a sudden change of direction causes the brain to rapidly move within the skull. The resultant bruising this causes can cause a temporary disruption of brain function – meaning the brain will not work as well as it is supposed to for a while — only 50% of patients with MTBI experience any symptoms. The appearance of symptoms is no cause for worry though, as it is normal. It is important to note that symptoms might only appear hours, even days, after the injury.

More than 85% of patients recover fully within one week, and 97% after one month. Age and health can influence the time to recovery. Most patients make a full recovery. In the UK, it was reported, 88% of all MTBI patients go back to full-time employment within three months. Only three to five percent of MTBI patients will suffer ongoing complications and difficulties with:

☐ Attention

☐ Concentration

☐ Short-term memory

☐ Planning and organizing tasks

☐ Keeping things in mind for periods of time

As a rule, patients generally find that their brain becomes slower. Most of these symptoms will clear up on its own because brain disruption is almost never permanent. Symptoms will be enhanced when the patient is tired, under pressure or worried about his/her condition.

Post-Concussive Syndrome

The post-concussive symptoms, also known as the *Post-Concussive Syndrome (PCS)*, are a part of the normal healing process and no cause for worry. Most of these symptoms will disappear without any treatment at all.

TABLE 1.4 SYMPTOMS OF POST-CONCUSSION SYNDROME

SYMPTOM	PREVALENCE
Attention deficit	71%
Confusion	57%
Depression	63%
Disrupted sleep	80%
Exhaustion	64%
Forgetfulness	59%
Headaches	59%
Impaired vision	45%
Moodiness	66%
Nervousness	58%
Sensitivity to Bright Light	40%
Vertigo	52%

When to return to the hospital?

When any of the following symptoms suddenly appear after a MTBI, it is of paramount importance to go back to the emergency room:

☐ Repeated Vomiting

☐ Worsening and constant headache

☐ Inability to stay awake

☐ Loss of consciousness

☐ Increased confusion, restlessness or agitation

☐ Convulsions

☐ Seizures

☐ Vertigo

☐ Difficulty walking

- ☐ Weakness
- ☐ Numbness
- ☐ Impaired vision

How to feel better?

Plenty of rest, relaxation and sleep will help heal the brain. Take it slow, and gradually return to old routines. Avoid demanding physical or mental activities and avoid alcohol. Do not return to sports and recreational activities before a thorough medical check-up and the green light from your health care professional.

CHAPTER 2

The First Few Days

DISORDERS OF CONSCIOUSNESS

After emergency treatment patients can be confronted by a variety of possible conditions and scenarios. To begin with, patients may suffer from altered levels of consciousness or disorders of consciousness (DOC). DOCs can be categorized as coma, vegetative state (VS), minimally conscious state (MCS) and Posttraumatic Confusional State (PTCS).

As a general rule, TBI will often result in the patient entering a comatose state for anything between a few days to several weeks. As the brainstem and the posterior part of the forebrain resume function, the patient will enter a VS state. Some patients may go directly into the VS without ever entering a comatose state.

COMA

Coma is a state of deep unconsciousness in which the eyes remain closed, and the patient cannot be aroused at all. Notable is the complete absence of any sign of a sleep-wake cycle. The JFK Coma Recovery Scale-Revised (CRS-R) is the most accurate clinical evaluation measure of disorders of consciousness. It assesses auditory, visual, verbal and motor functions together with communication and arousal levels.

There is no reliable way to predict how long a person will remain in a coma, nor what the long-term effects of the brain injury that caused the coma, will be. People have individual recovery trajectories, and no two injuries of the brain are the same. However, it seems self-evident that a rapid recovery from a coma will be considered a very good sign.

Some people though, after recovering from a coma quickly, might experience some serious problems at a later stage, while some patients might remain in a coma for months and months before making a full recovery.

Despite this, the length of a coma is one of the most reliable predictors of the severity of long-term symptoms after TBI. The longer the coma, the more likely there will be lasting problems.

VEGETATIVE STATE (VS)

A VS can be described as the absence of any behavioral evidence of self-awareness or awareness of the environment when there is evidence of the restoration of the reticular activating system (eyes are opening, or patient is awake). In these circumstances, there is a complete absence of purposeful responses to visual stimuli, touch or unpleasant prodding (pinprick), and an apparent lack of understanding of language or the expression of language.

The outdated use of Persistent VS and Permanent VS are discouraged now, simply because these terms not only describe a level of consciousness but also imply a prognosis, which might be quite misleading.

Even so, statistically the period of sustained VS is relevant for prognosis. Victims who remain in a VS for more than one year after suffering a TBI has a lowered probability of recovering awareness.

However, *miracles* happen very often.

According to studies more than 20% of patients in a VS for between 14 and 28 months after injury onset will progress to a minimally conscious state *or will regain consciousness*.

Outcomes for younger patients are on average, more favorable.

Patients who remain in VS can live for five years, and even ten years and miracles revive some of these patients years later, too.

Functional neuroimaging can help to identify covert cognitive functioning in patients with VS by demonstrating physiological reactions (such as changes in regional blood flow) to environmental stimuli. Functional MRI can detect brain activity by detecting the blood oxygen level dependent signal, and studies showed that patients in which fMRI detected brain activity in this way, almost all of them eventually processed to at least a minimally conscious state during the observational period.

MINIMALLY CONSCIOUS STATE (MCS)

Despite MCS being a severely altered state of consciousness, in this state minimal but undeniable behavioral evidence of self-awareness or environmental awareness is demonstrated. In MCs reactions to stimuli occur, but inconsistently. It is, however, clear and present enough to be reproducible and sustained long enough to be differentiated from normal reflexive behavior.

When a patient is asked to follow simple commands or responds with gestural or verbal yes or no affirmations, purposeful behavior or even intelligible verbalization, a diagnosis of MCS can be inferred.

MCS has to be carefully differentiated from coma or VS. This can be done by carefully recording the presence of behavioral features absent from the same. MCS patients will display some signs of cognitive processing and pain perception, while patients in VS do not respond to any noxious stimuli.

In MCS, interactive communication is possible. Verbalization, writing and yes/no responses occur and sometimes augmented communication devices can be used. Before the functional use of objects can be inferred the patient has to be able to use two different objects appropriately. Functional outcome for MCS patients is significantly better than for those in VS.

It is important to take note that for patients who suffered TBI and are in either a VS or MCS, **treatment with amantadine has been shown to improve functional recovery.** The use of amantadine should as a matter of course be considered for this population.

POSTTRAUMATIC CONFUSIONAL STATE (PTCS)

PTCS is a relatively new distinction of another disorder of consciousness. According to modern scholars, PTCS is a distinct state that has to be differentiated from MCS, and this occurs when there is a reemergence of a reliable yes/no communication system or when the patient succeeds in using (two or more) familiar objects in a functional manner.[ii]

During the PTCS the patient will experience and demonstrate temporal and spatial disorientation, distractibility, anterograde amnesia (the inability to remember any new information), impaired judgment, perceptual disturbance, sleep disorder, emotional lability, and restlessness.

According to Stuss the cognitive disturbances during PTCS are more important than any amnesia, which is considered concomitant at best.

Confusion and agitation, anxiety and distress will be marked. This can be accompanied by disinhibited behavior such as sexual inappropriate displays and swearing. Periods of unusual quiet and docility, neediness or childlike behavior can follow, and patients might wander off, even try to walk away despite broken limbs. Sometimes the patient will not be able to recognize anyone.

Again, the length of the PTCS is important. The longer it lasts, the more severe the brain injuries tend to be, and the more severe the long-term effects are expected to be. PTCS lasting longer than 24 hours are usually considered to be severe.

DISORDERS OF MOVEMENT

The most common movement disorder seen in patients, who suffered TBI, is a tremor. Posttraumatic movement disorders can be transient or persistent and can include tremor and dystonia (muscle spasms and unnatural posture). Younger patients will often show the longest latency (period after the TBI before the movement disorder starts), and they seem to show a greater likelihood of suffering from generalized dystonia.

Movement disorders like ataxia are very hard to treat. Ataxia, a loss of full control of bodily movements, can sometimes be treated by beta-blockers and stereotactic surgery, but the results are usually disappointing. Severe upper limb ataxia can even make it difficult to feed yourself, but - without limiting the ability to walk, for example.

Following TBI two main types of movement disorder are normally seen. In the first place, there is a loss of mobility – hemiparesis (paralysis of one side of the body) or quadriparesis (weakness of all four limbs of the body) and in second place, involuntary movement (tremor, dystonia, etc.). Patients with severe quadriparesis might be so affected that they cannot even roll over in bed.

Dyskinesia, the insuppressible automatic movements of the limbs is another form of involuntary movement disorder that occurs in patients with TBI.

Muscle bulk in traumatic brain injury patients often atrophies as a result of prolonged coma or immobility. Muscle tone abnormalities may also result from TBI. Spasticity might result in (increased resistance to passive movements) as well as rigidity, while paratonia (inability to relax muscles voluntarily) also occurs.

Further motor control impairments might present as weakness, decreased coordination, impaired initiation, and motor restlessness. Balance impairments will present in up to 60% of TBI patients.

Movement disorders will present in between 13% and 66% of patients after TBI.

In one of the largest studies of survivors of TBI, posttraumatic movement disorders persisted in only 12.2% of survivors.

The most common movement disorder that persisted was tremor, followed by dystonia.
The less severe the injury of the brain, the less prevalent movement disorders appears to be.

In mild to moderate TBI survivors, posttraumatic movement disorders were reported in only 10.1% and persisted in only 2.6% of cases.

Movement disorders are classified into:

- hyperkinetic disorders (slowness and the paucity of movement), which includes tremor, dystonia, ballism (jerking or flinging of an extremity) and
- chorea (unpredictable dance-like movements), tics and
- tourettism (semi-voluntary repetitive movements or vocalizations),
- myoclonus (Sudden shock-like movements) and
- hyperekplexia (exaggerated startle response) and
- akathisia (inner sense of restlessness) and

- hypokinetic disorders, described as Parkinsonism characterized by rigidity, resting tremor and postural instability. The onset of Parkinsonism is normally within a few months after the TBI.

STATE OF MIND

Family members of TBI patients go through severe emotional distress. Not only are they expected to make continuous decisions about their loved one's care and treatment, but they also experience a sense of loss and insecurity about the situation and the chances of survival of the TBI patient. They are also placed in a situation where they must accept increased responsibility for the loved one's physical, emotional and financial wellbeing.

Caregivers often experience severe psychological distress, and this is normally exposed when they display a high level of denial about the injuries, social withdrawal, irritability and concentration problems, as well as anger towards the TBI patient.

When this happens, it is a regrettable dilution not only of the caregiver's quality of life; it also impacts the patient's life negatively. If the caregiver is negative, unrealistic, unhelpful and not assertive enough, this has a negative impact on the patient, and the patient will experience greater difficulty to escape mental and psychological distress right after the TBI when negative emotions can create more havoc in his nervous system.

Some strategies can be followed by caregivers to prevent themselves from becoming emotionally-burdened to the extent that they cannot carry and uplift the patient in her time of need. Caregivers must find the time to talk to family members about their fears and feelings, and they must make a point of not becoming socially-isolated by just focusing on hospital visits. Do not withdraw socially!

Make time to engage in activities that bring great enjoyment, albeit reading, music or taking long walks with the dog – whatever you do, it will help you cope with the traumatic events.

By educating yourself on brain injury, it becomes easier to accept things and get on with the process of living life, for yourself and your injured loved one. Getting some exercise during the early stages of post-trauma when your loved one is starting to recover and needs you there, is a proven method to improve your mood and your emotional endurance.

During this phase, the patient will need a lot of positive affirmations before she is able to find peace and start accepting her new life situation.

No matter what my symptoms, my health is improving every second
I am thankful for the healing that is restoring my body
I am willing to accept what happened and I choose to overcome
My body will follow my mind, and my mind will demand full recovery
I am more than my injuries. I am more than my pain. I am a healing force
Miracles come to those who believe, and I believe
If I can visualize it, I can achieve it, and I can see myself become whole again

It is often the small things that matter, and every individual will have their own individualized approach, but some examples of the types of positive affirmation that will mean a lot to the patient during the very early stages of the TBI follow below.

- Gingerly remind the loved one that he is safe
- Also, remind him where he is from, time to time
- Bring family pictures and personal items to the hospital from home to make him feel comfortable
- Stay with him and help him keep pace with time

- Help him to keep calm
- Keep noise levels low around him
- Do not allow more than one or two visitors at his bedside at any one time

Small tokens of love and nurture like these will provide emotional support and encouragement to the loved one during the early stages of TBI. Being positive and supportive will also provide positive reinforcement to the caregiver, and this will help prevent negativity and despair both ways.

Coping with the flights of denial and the temper outbursts of the patient during the first few days can be cumbersome. Some easy strategies can help a lot towards calming the loved one down and preventing aggression.

- Understanding creates acceptance. Once it is understood that the loved one's anger and irritability is due to the TBI, caregivers will no longer take outbursts of aggression personally
- Under no circumstances should caregivers argue or engage with a loved one during outbursts. The loved one should be allowed to act out and cool down before taking any kind of contrary view.
- Caregivers should never be tempted to preserve peace and quiet by giving in to the loved one's angry demands and outbursts.
- Do a post-mortem after the temper attack. Discuss the outburst calmly with the loved one and try to figure out the source of the anger in a mutual and calm manner.

- Rules of engagement should be used to set parameters. The loved one should clearly understand that despite his injuries and difficult situation, he is still not permitted to hurt or threaten or scream at anybody. Reinforce this line of communication by refusing to respond or even talk to the loved one during his temper tantrum.

DISCHARGE PLAN

A planned and organized discharge from the hospital decreases the chance that TBI patients will be readmitted to the hospital again. If the discharge is arranged well, recovery is speeded up when all the required medicines are prescribed beforehand and given at the right times and at the correct dosages. This is the epoch of short hospitalization. Hospitals are increasingly pressured into releasing patients "quicker and sicker," and this makes proper discharge planning critical for the patient's continuous recovery. It has been reported that close to 20% of Medicare patients will be readmitted to the hospital within 20 days after discharge, while as much as 40% of all senior patients will suffer from medication errors when they go home.

It is never too soon to start developing the discharge plan for a TBI patient. Within the first few days after admission, it is already appropriate to start planning the process. The discharge for these patients should rather be seen as a transition into a real-world scenario without interrupting treatment or discontinuing recovery. Far from it. From day one, the discharge plan is slowly formulated and constantly redrafted as things change and develop.

PRE-PLANNING

During this early planning stage, the family and caregivers have to consult with the hospital in order to tailor the plan for their specific needs and circumstances by considering the following important factors:

a. Access: How easy will it be to get into the family home if the patient cannot walk when they arrive home and has to be brought in either in a hospital type bed or wheelchair?

b. Are there any suggested community activities the family and the patient can become involved in to aid the recovery and rehabilitation process?

c. Does the family have the required financial resources to provide care and support for the patient and irrespective of the answer to this question; are there any public benefits the family is eligible for?

d. Supervision: How much patient supervision will be required, and who will take responsibility for this task?

e. Support: Which family members will be available to help and support the patient, and what exactly does it take to "help & support" this injured family member when they arrive home?

f. The patient will most likely require medical treatment, nursing care, and therapy after being discharged to the family residence. How will this be accomplished and by whom? Will there be a residential program or outpatient therapy program available?

g. What type of transport will be required to move the patient from the hospital to the family residence?

AS THE DISCHARGE DATE APPROACHES

Every patient discharge is a unique event, but some general aspects need to be considered for every unique discharge. The patient has to be provided with proper documentation and information if the discharge is to be seamless and not disruptive.

Patients should be provided with and actively supported in the effort, to put together a complete discharge summary including the following:[iii]

a.   Active problems at discharge

b.   Carer information

c.   Comprehensive and reconciled medication list

d.   Dates of admission and discharge

e.   Details of all the doctors involved with the patient's care

f.   Discharge diagnosis

g.   Follow up arrangements

h.   Information on drugs started and stopped in the hospital and the reasons for this.

i.   Prognosis

j.   Reason for hospitalization

k.   Treatment received while in hospital

INFORMATION THE PATIENT AND CAREGIVERS NEED BEFORE DISCHARGE

a.   Assistance. What level of assistance will be required once the patient arrives home, and who will take responsibility for this?

b.   Date of discharge?

c.   Did the hospital provide the patient with a discharge teaching sheet?

d. Equipment. What equipment will be needed when the patient arrives home and who will acquire and set up the equipment?

e. Exercise program. Does the patient require a home therapy/ exercise program, and who will provide the details for this?

f. Family doctor. Does the patient need to be visited by a family doctor after arriving home?

g. Follow-up appointments. Will the patient need follow-up appointments and who will make the appointments?

h. Insurance. Who will arrange the patient's medical insurance affairs and who will provide the doctors and hospital with the required details and paperwork?

i. Medical certificates. Will, the patient, requires medical certificates for insurance or work-related reasons, and who will supply the same?

j. Medication changes. Under what conditions and for which reasons can/must the patient change the medication taken?

k. Pre-injury medication. Can the patient restart or continue taking medication and supplements taken before the TBI?

l. Prescriptions. Does the patient need medical prescriptions before leaving the hospital?

m. Prognosis. What is the patient's prognosis?

n. Questions. Who can be called after discharge, if the patient has questions or needs information?

o. Restrictions. Are there any specific restrictions on the patient once discharged?

WHAT HOSPITALS OFFER TBI PATIENTS

This is not a single question with a single answer. The medical marketplace is diverse, and facilities compete with one another to provide TBI patient care. As such, the product offered is very diverse.

In broad terms, hospitals offer specialized treatment and specialized equipment. Equipment offered can range from basic standing frames, augmented communication devices and iPad technology to sophisticated devices that provide electrical stimulation to promote motor recruitment, improve mobility and increase the functional use of the limbs, to training equipment that address gait performance and increased mobility. Some hospitals even provide working facility dogs that work as members of the medical team to aid the patients with little tasks like switching off the lights or retrieving fallen items, all the while providing love, comfort, and support to patients.

The range of specialized treatments is vast, diverse and almost unique to every institution. Some hospitals offer home evaluations (before discharge), memory aids, and advanced pharmacological and therapeutic interventions to manage a variety of subsequent conditions and more.

Some typical services can be listed:

    a.   Aphasia and cognitive therapy programs

    b.   Board certified physical medicine and rehabilitation physicians and nurses specializing in rehabilitation

    c.   Brain injury education and support groups

    d.   Brain injury residential programs for patients for patients ready for independent living.

    e.   Clinical-team conferences to discuss patient care and progress

f. Community re-integration trips

g. Continuous communication with qualified physicians

h. Exercise programs and safe support equipment

i. Hours of therapy (physical, occupational, speech, and others) every day of the week.

j. Intensive inpatient rehabilitation

k. Neurobehavioral programs

l. Neuro-optometry Consults

m. Neuropsychological testing

n. Outpatient brain injury specialty clinics offer comprehensive evaluation and treatment services.

o. Outpatient services at day hospitals and community rehabilitation programs to assist and aid recovery of patients in real-world settings in home and community environments

p. Physician-directed patient services

q. State-of-the-art medical and rehabilitation facilities

For treatment in the early stages of recovery from TBI, hospital inpatient rehabilitation services should get priority. This is especially true when there is evidence of notable behavioral, cognitive or physical difficulties after TBI. The overall goal of inpatient rehabilitation is to improve the patient's condition to such a degree that she can be discharged to the least restrictive setting possible, preferably to her home. According to research, the median length of hospital stay for TBI patients is 18 days.

WHAT NURSING FACILITIES AND NURSING HOMES OFFER TBI PATIENTS?

Patients are normally discharged to nursing homes or skilled nursing facilities when they suffered severe TBI, if they no longer need acute medical care as provided by a hospital, but are not ready for participation in outpatient rehabilitation, yet, or if the progress they made during inpatient treatment, slows down before they are ready to be discharged to their homes yet. These facilities are their best choice at this point.

Many nursing homes and skilled nursing facilities do not specialize in the treatment and rehabilitation of TBI specifically, but some do.

Nursing facilities and nursing homes that offer specialized care and support for TBI patients in a less clinical and more communal environment are often housed on beautiful grounds offering magnificent amenities, all depending on the patient's budget of course.

The communal approach encourages social interaction and engagement through arranged activities and participation in educational and wellness programs, as well as excursions into the surrounding community.

Recreational activities can include exercise, swimming pools, and adult education programs.

On a functional level, these facilities provide daily living assistance (clothing, hygiene, and grooming) as well as the provision of meals (or meal preparation assistance for those who so prefer). Skill building and pro-social interaction are developed, and money management is taught and supported. Supervised community integration is provided alongside medication and behavior assistance.

Medical and rehabilitation care is provided by qualified nurses, neuropsychologists, certified nursing, and medical assistants, dieticians, case managers, and activity coordinators and trained residential aides providing crises intervention.

GOAL SETTING

In broad terms, the goal of rehabilitation after TBI is to improve the patient's functioning at home and in society to such an extent that the patient can adapt to their disabilities and to adopt the required environmental modifications to make the patient's everyday life as easy and comfortable as possible.

To facilitate these rehabilitation goals, the TBI patients and their families must work together to select the most appropriate rehabilitation environment. There are so many options that it can be quite a daunting task to really select the best setting for this purpose.

a. Home-based rehabilitation

b. Hospital outpatient rehabilitation

c. Inpatient rehabilitation centers

d. Comprehensive day care rehabilitation centers

e. Supported living programs

f. Independent living centers

g. Club-house programs

h. School-based programs (children)

i. Others

Without due consultation and collaboration of the patient, the family, and the rehabilitation team members, an informed choice will just not be possible. There is a consensus that for TBI patients, individualized rehabilitation programs need to be developed based on specific individual needs and that this should be modified as time goes by, according to changing needs.

It is recommended that moderately or severely injured patients opt for rehabilitation that draws from the skills of multiple specialists. Individual programs utilizing physical & occupational or speech therapy, physical medicine, psychiatry, and social support and more, should be developed.

Healthcare workers have to engage patients and their families during the goal-setting process in order to understand the individual's life context and to respond to their questions and concerns. They should endeavor to clarify the individual and the families understanding of the brain injury, as well as on their likely progress. It is essential that all the parties should be given ample opportunity to share their views on the future before a collaborative goal setting can be optimized.

Setting appropriate goals, meaningful to the patient and his family is a critical component of care and will shape the person's future participation in meaningful activities as well as their discharge destination.

One of the options open to patients, when rehabilitation goals and destinations are considered, is outpatient rehabilitation services. Patients can be referred to the same directly from the hospital, or when they are discharged from inpatient rehabilitation. Outpatient services might include psychological services and various forms of therapy.

Patients with TBI often have real difficulty in articulating goals, and often revert to stating goals in very broad or general terms, like "I want to go home" or "I want to get strong." To make this easier, both family members and healthcare workers need to assist by breaking the goals down by asking for more detail, by making suggestions and by engaging each other.

In order to set realistic goals, the patient and her family have to be very clear on the degree of recovery to expect and how to achieve the greatest outcome. Healthcare workers have to provide significant direction and support to clarify the treatment focus. From their side, patients identify goals that facilitate transfer to rehabilitation or discharge into the community.

The ideal goal setting outcome would be a combination of the therapist led goals setting and the goals set by the patient and his family. Once the therapist has provided enough information about the steps required for recovery, the family and the patient can engage and decide the goals they wish to pursue, in terms of therapy and environment, in order to optimize recovery.

WEEK ONE AFTER DISCHARGE: WHAT TO EXPECT

The move back home might be exciting for the patient and family members, but it certainly is not stress-free. When the loved one returns, it is often very clear very quickly that no amount of preparation could actually succeed in preparing caregivers for what lies ahead. Normal life for most people is based on independence, some time alone, work, school, volunteering and driving, doing your own household chores, living socially and choosing what to do and when to do it. When a TBI patient returns home, almost none of the above is possible for her or for the caregiver family.

It is often reported that the patient's condition or recovery actually takes a few steps back during the first week or two at home. This happens because the patient needs more time than a healthy person would, to adapt to the changed environment. This is a fairly common occurrence and should not be a cause of worry if it remains contained to the first few days.

No matter how much planning was done before the patient arrived back home, the first week will require constant changes and adaptations to the environment to make the transition as smooth as possible. Even the skills that the patient might have acquired during rehabilitation so far might not transfer easily to the home setting without a lot of reinforcement and support from family members.

For a TBI patient, structure and routine make life easier to comprehend and control. Everything in the patient's life has to be scheduled and routinized. Over time, the strict structure may be loosened, and a more flexible scenario might develop, but absolutely not at the beginning.

Especially in the beginning, family caregivers might be completely overwhelmed by all that they have to do, and their energy might be sapped very quickly. Time management skills will be required to prioritize tasks, and all the members of the family will have to pitch in to get the thing going.

Small thing that makes time management and scheduling very difficult during the first week is the incessant phone calls that often come in from all the friends and family. Everyone will want updates and communicate their well-wishes to the patient and the family, and this can be very perilous if there is a lot of pressure in the home to adapt to the changing circumstances.

The first week will show the caregivers for the first time, what tasks and chores they will have to complete on a daily and weekly basis, and lists of tasks can immediately be made to create routines and to make smooth instinctive action possible.

During the first week, all the tasks that have to be done might be overwhelming. Food preparation, housework and transportation and management of family finances are everyday tasks. Care tasks like arranging and keeping medical appointments, supervision, personal hygiene and medical and nursing care never stops. Emotional support, recreation and legal, educational and work arrangements are also recurrent and have to be handled continuously.

During the first week, more home modifications that are required will be identified and has to be done as soon as possible to make life bearable for the patient and the caregivers. Caregivers will also have to cope with assistive devices that were installed or supplied. They will have to know how to use them, and what for. This could include special beds, timers, special phones and more.

The most difficult and daunting task caregivers will have to master during the first week, is to manage the patient's medications. Just to have the right medicines available at the right times, is often a huge undertaking. Prescriptions have to be picked up, and a medication log has to be kept to track all treatments. All of this can be made much harder if the family is experiencing financial hardships due to the medical and treatment costs or loss of income.

One of the most difficult things to adapt to, for family members, is to get used to the changes, albeit permanent or not, in the personality and temperament of the patient. Patients will often be frustrated, angry, and their likely memory loss can make it almost impossible to find any continuity at the beginning when they arrive home. Getting to know the new - albeit impermanent – family member can elicit a lot of sadness and emotion in caregivers. These changes will be amplified during the first week or so when the patient comes back home for the first time, and family members inevitably compare the old person to the new, damaged person home for rehabilitation.

CHAPTER 03

Early recovery

OUTPATIENT REHABILITATION THERAPIES

For most TBI patients that have been discharged home, years of therapy and rehabilitation will follow. It is entirely possible to return home and still receive the full complement of therapy and treatments available from a TBI day hospital or outpatient program. Sometimes these facilities are not part of a hospital outpatient program as such but are formed by the aggregation of various therapy programs and practitioners at a specific location. These facilities are often more than adequate for the less-severe TBI patient that might only require specific rehabilitation and treatment that can be accessed either in the traditional hospital outpatient department or via the office or home-based treatments.

For severe TBI patients, some hospitals offer one-stop facilities provided by outpatient clinics that employ nurse practitioners, rehab nurses and rehab technicians that work with the outpatient therapy team. These clinics aid in the development of home programs for the patient and their caregivers and family members.

Outpatient therapy is often a long-term process that will last much longer than inpatient treatment. The team of outpatient healthcare providers will coordinate and develop a set of goals for the rehabilitation of the patient to optimize the patient's recovery. It is important for the family members and caregivers to closely coordinate with the health care providers to ensure that they not only understand these goals but that they remain realistic about what can be achieved over a given period of time.

Generally speaking, outpatient rehabilitation will involve at least two to three sessions per week. During these sessions, the TBI patients might be required to do up to one hour each of physical, occupational and speech therapy with the goal of improving the patient's life by making him/her more independent, improving their skills for a return to school or work, and allowing them more freedom to participate in in recreational activities of their preference.

PHYSICAL THERAPY

As mentioned above, most TBI patients will require up to three therapy sessions per week, and these might include various types of therapy for an hour each, all in series.

Physical therapists treat disorders of the human body by physical means rather than by prescribing drugs. At the beginning of the treatment, the physical therapist will work in conjunction with the medical team treating the TBI patient, especially when assessing the treatment objectives for the patient. One of their functions is to prevent the deterioration of the patient's condition that might result from their existent injuries.

These physical therapists (PT) are specialists in human movement dysfunctions and trained to treat the patient in order to strengthen their physical abilities. For this purpose, they use therapeutic exercise, electrical stimulation, heat and cold and the application and provision of devices such as braces. They achieve their aims by helping the patient to improve their coordination, endurance, and impairments.

The PT will diagnose impairments in the patient before deciding on treatment options. The PT evaluation will include a study of the patient's posture while sitting and standing, as well as inspecting the way the TBI patient holds her arms and neck.

The patient's range of motion is of particular importance to the PT. The PT will measure the active and passive range of motion of the patient at every point in the body where the patient experience pain or discomfort. Apart from range of movement, the quality of movement will be measured. To treat the patient for headaches, and even to prevent the onset of headaches, the PT will look specifically at the temporal mandibular joint for dysfunctions (pain and stiffness related to the movements of the jaw of the patient).

Further assessments will be made to inspect neurological (motor/ sensory/balance) symptoms, and palpation (touching and feeling the patient's muscles to examine the size, consistency, texture, and tenderness of a muscle or body part) especially to help identify joint dysfunctions.

OCCUPATIONAL THERAPY

Whereas physical therapy is mainly aimed at treating disorders of the body, especially movement dysfunctions by using exercise and other forms of physical intervention to improve the patient's mobility, occupation therapy is focused on the skills required for the job of living. After a TBI, patients may be impaired from doing the things that are important to their life and functioning. The inability to care for themselves, the inability to work or to participate in hobbies, sport or family events, might all contribute to a patient's failing sense of self and belief in the future. Occupational therapists intervene at this point by teaching the patient new skills and strategies – new ways of doing things, by adapting and redesigning the materials and equipment used, and by adapting the patient's environment to negotiate flexibility from employers, re-organizing work and living space, and by educating and training caregivers and peers about the patient's abilities and impairments.

On a more technical level, it can be said that the occupational therapist makes a comparison between a patient's capacity and her actual performance, and then does almost the same thing by comparing the patient's performance with his environment. After gathering all the required data, the occupational therapist will endeavor to equalize the patient's performance to her capacity and to improve their performance above their capacity by changing their environment.

SPEECH THERAPY

After TBI many patients display severe cognitive and communication impairments. Many patients have serious trouble swallowing, and speech and language impairments might torment the patient and their loved ones & caregivers. Individual treatment programs are developed by speech therapists to intervene and help the patient to improve or even recover their speech, language abilities and swallowing problems.

The speech therapist will assess the patient for various signs and symptoms, including poor concentration, confusion, disorientation and the repetition of a specific word, phrase or gesture, verbal confabulation (reporting events that never happened due to memory impairment) and for the presence of inappropriate comments or behavior in social contexts, and lack of verbal reasoning skills.

Therapy might result in the provision and training for the use of an augmented communication device, or the improvement of memory, reasoning, and problem-solving skills.

PSYCHOLOGICAL THERAPY

During recovery from TBI, more than 40% of patients will suffer from agitated behavior, and at least 33% will display high levels of aggression. Some research indicates that up to 70% of TBI patients will suffer from irritability and agitation for up to 15-years after their injuries. Some of the most common behavioral problems TBI patients suffer from include inappropriate social communication skills, the strange inability to stop ongoing behavior, poor impulse control, and emotional-availability, as well as impaired behavioral regulation.

TBI patients will benefit from psychological intervention by therapists for the alleviation and management of these symptoms, and they will greatly benefit from psychological therapy even in the absence of behavioral problems just to manage their adjustment disorder that most likely comes with the enormous situational depression and despair that usually accompanies the disruptive life changes that TBI patients have to adjust to.

SCHEDULING

People suffering from brain injuries need even more sleep than those without injuries need. It is normal for TBI patients to need more than ten hours of sleep per night, and early after the injuries, they might even need naps throughout the day too. Sleep and rest are crucial for the brain to recover, and any form of over-exertion is perilous and can cause recovery to slow down, or even stop altogether.

The TBI patient's life has to be formally structured for her to seize the day and control her life. Even sleep and rest has to be scheduled in order to allow for rest and sleep before the patient actually becomes tired. Once tired, it may take the TBI several days to recoup their strength again.

To prevent burnouts and preserve the integrity of the schedule it has to be flexible yet fixed. If the patient becomes tired, it will take him longer to complete the scheduled task. The more fatigued the patient becomes, the more effort he will have to put in. This can cause frustration and – of course – exhaustion. It is imperative that patients, especially those with type-A personalities who are really driven, must be coached to slow down in situations like this. It is not about finishing the task, for TBI patients it is actually all about the journey. Speed kills, as they say.

One of the most important considerations, when a schedule is designed, is the dire need for routine and consistency. Whether it is for medical treatment or for personal hygiene, meals or rest, the body and the mind must receive what is anticipated. Mealtimes, the mind, and the body, anticipate food. It is actually a shock to the system if a massage and some physiotherapy arrive in lieu of food. Nothing must ever be erratic; everything must be totally consistent.

Along with fixed schedules, it is advisable to develop checklists - a checklist for leaving the house; another one for returning home and yet another list of medications and recreation, and so on. To add to the list, make a checklist for a life well-planned, and use it to supplement the clarity of the plan and checklist. Every single task or activity should have a carefully written objective and a set of goals to be achieved. This can help to stimulate memory and will help the patient with continuity if she is interrupted or has to go back to the task later on.

ENROLLING IN REHABILITATION

As a matter of course, patients with TBI have special rehabilitation needs. A case in point, some symptoms of brain injury mirror the symptoms of depression. If treatment for the symptoms of depression is sought from a practitioner, who is not specifically equipped to treat depression *in TBI patients*, TBI symptoms like low energy and a lack of concentration might be treated inappropriately for someone suffering from TBI injuries.

In order to make a really informed decision about the extent of the patient's needs for rehabilitation, and to figure out a rehabilitation strategy and objectives, it is advisable to contact a social worker or psychologist to assess the functional independence of the patient. This is achieved by using the Functional Independence Measure to measure the patient's self-care skills, toilet, bladder and bowel management, transfers and locomotion, communication and cognition. These are the functions that will ultimately need intervention through rehabilitation. The lower the patient's score on this assessment, the more rehabilitation and assistance will be needed by him. The measure is also used over time to measure the patient's progress over time.

Another useful assessment is the Craig Handicap Assessment and Reporting Technique that helps to assess the functional outcome later in the process of rehabilitation and measures social and community participation.

There is a big difference between hope, beliefs and grand optimism, believing in miracles (which do happen sometimes) and superhuman results brought on by an iron will, and such. These are existential and spiritual goals, and it should not be confused with the goals of rehabilitation. Rehabilitation goals are predicated by informed visions of what might be achieved when specific treatment options are selected from the list of available options, and these options are often a function of the available financial resources, the clinical assessment of the patient's injuries, the stage of recovery the patient is in at the moment, the dedication of both the patient, her caregivers, and family as well as her health care providers. It is a complicated and involved process that necessitates the involvement of all the parties.

Some writers distinguish between active and passive goals. A passive goal is aimed at the facilitation of care, for example, keeping hygiene standards very high, never allowing the patient to remain immobile for long periods of time, and avoiding sores and muscle spasms this way, and increasing the comfort level of a wheelchair by adjusting the patient's position to maximize comfort and pressure on muscles and skin.

Active goals are for attempts to improve the patient's active functioning, to gain more function through intervention and therapy. It is very important to keep the expectations realistic, and by assessing even the smallest improvements as big victories. It is often underestimated how much even the minutest improvement in function can mean to the patients of TBI.

Realism and effective goal setting cannot exist outside a team approach. Only if the family, caregivers and a team of professionals with a deep understanding of the patient's potential for recovery and knowledge of the potential positive impact of various possible interventions, can develop a shared vision for rehabilitation, will realistic goals be decided on, and actually achieved.

The more severe the TBI is the more important the participation of the family, and caregivers will be. In severe cases, feedback from the patient must be used when goal development takes place, but the feedback has to be viewed within the context of family goals and the patient's strengths and limits. The lower the patient's level of awareness, the more careful goal development has to be.

For those with severe TBI, goal setting will have to be an ever-growing focus on passive goals- that is, on methods that can address methods of compensation for the difficulties the patient face in a functional sense.

On another level, it is of extreme importance that the family and caregivers understand and support the consensus about the treatment and the goals decided upon. In this sense, the attitude of the family in terms of the goals is of critical importance, that is, their real beliefs about short-and long-term goals will inform the patient beliefs and will set the standard for the whole process. For this reason, the development of goals has to include the family and caregivers in a comprehensive and real way.

Put differently, the family and caregiver control the environment, resources, and access to the patient. Any goal development that excludes those in control of the patient's world will be doomed to fail.

CAREGIVING AT HOME

TRANSITION TO ORAL FEEDING

Before a patient can transition from tube-feeding to oral feeding, that is, before she can start taking food by mouth, she has to meet five conditions. First-off, the patient must be medically stable. Needless to say, the brain injury must be improved enough for the patient's eyes to remain open and for the patient to be able to respond to painful stimulation. These are more or less self-evident. If a tracheostomy tube is still present, it has to be either small or fitted with a cuff that can be deflated. The most important thing to double check before a patient can start taking food by mouth is the ability to swallow. Many TBI patients develop severe difficulty swallowing, and it is advisable to invite an occupational therapist to come and assess the patient's ability to swallow and take food by mouth before transitioning to oral feeding. Another crucial element that has to be 100% present is the patient's coughing reflex. If the patient's coughing reflex is strong enough, the airway into the lungs will be protected, and oral feeding will be safe.

As soon as the patient's swallowing and cough reflexes are up to standard, foods of specific consistencies will be provided to the patient to mirror the level of recovery of the swallowing ability of the patient. For a start, liquids will be provided, and slowly thickened until soft and blended foods will replace the liquids. The occupational therapist will gradually allow the addition of new and different foods depending on the progress made. For some patients, supplemental feeding via a feeding tube might be required to optimize nutrition while the patient relearns how to swallow normally.

If the patient shows any signs of chewing difficulty or finds it difficult to move food to the back of the mouth or to swallow, care should be taken. Further, if the patient tends to cough or choke often, or develops a wet-sounding voice with congestion in the chest – or becomes tired or short of breath while eating, swallowing difficulties might be hampering the patient more than anticipated, and an occupational therapist has to be consulted.

From the caregiver or family's side, it will help a lot if they learned the steps to follow for safe eating and made sure that they were present during meal times. Also, slowing the pace of eating down will make it easier for the patient to swallow at her own leisure, and to swallow only when it is safe to do so.

Speed is the enemy. Reminding the patient consistently to eat and drink slowly, and especially not to speak until the mouth is clear of food, will go a long way towards making things easier for the patient.

SELF-AWARENESS AND INSIGHT

Cheryle Sullivan writes that TBI patients often use huge amounts of energy during the day irrespective of how self-aware they are, trying not to appear brain-damaged. This, she writes, happens because of the patient's burning desire to appear as normal as possible. Sullivan's revelation introduces us to the conundrum of brain injury. Pretending and fighting to appear more "normal" or "less brain-damaged" than they think they really are is actually an example of the type of self-unawareness many TBI patients suffer from.

It is very important that TBI patients realize early on that they are human beings, not, as Sullivan explains, "*human doings.*" When they lose the ability to do the things they used to do, they simply lose what they used to do, not what they are. The insight that "we" are not brain injured – we are persons with brain injuries, is crucial before a TBI injury can embark on a rehabilitation program.

A lack of awareness – or put differently – unawareness (anosognosia), is a thing apart from denial. Patients who suffer from severe "unawareness" are not using defense mechanisms to deny their problems to themselves, and the world. These patients are actually unaware that any problems exist. This can be both dangerous and an impairment to rehabilitation.

If the patient seems completely unconcerned, acting as if absolutely nothing is amiss, there *is* a reason to worry. These patients might insist that they can do everything just as well as always, or they might insist that they can and want to do some things that you certainly know they cannot. This might become obvious when the patient takes the position that neither her doctor nor her caregivers have a clue what they are doing, or when they start to blame those around them for the things they cannot do, the presence of anosognosia should be inferred until further notice. This condition might put the patient at extreme risk, and it might cause them to use power tools that they cannot control or attempt activities they cannot achieve, and this might lead to serious injuries and harm.

FECAL AND URINARY INCONTINENCE

Injuries to the frontal lobes of the brain often cause the loss of cortical control over bowel and bladder. Research shows that more than 62% of patients with frontal lobe injuries develop urinary incontinence. This is concomitant with an increased risk of urinary tract infection and skin ulcer development.

Urinary incontinence can be treated and managed by following scheduled and timed voiding programs and by the use of anticholinergic agents.[iv] Similarly, bowel movements can be managed with a timed voiding schedule, fiber supplementation, and consistent hydration. Stool softeners and suppositories can be used moderately and under medical supervision.

Patients who are impaired and cannot control their bowl emptying voluntarily or recognize the fullness of their bowls, or those who cannot walk to the bathroom or ask for assistance, or those who cannot consume enough food, fluid, and fiber, or cannot plan activities anymore and consequently cannot reach the bathroom in time, will need assistance to manage their bowel function. The same goes for urinary impairment.

COMMUNICATION TOOLS

Anything that can aid communication can be considered a communication tool, whether it is a drumbeat, smoke signal or tapping Morse code against a wall. However, for the benefit of the TBI patient, it is safer to stick to the conventional rather than the exotic. The modern mobile device, or cell phone, is the most powerful communication tool ever conceptualized. For a TBI patient, the mobile phone with all the apps that are available can be a miracle-providing-machine. It might be warranted to supply the TBI patient with a headset to aid hearing and conversations, and it will be precautious to supply both an old-fashioned landline and a mobile phone.

Old-fashioned equipment like answering machines and even desktop or laptop computers are almost redundant as communication tools for TBI patients. Modern mobile phones and various models of tablets will suffice and are much easier for the TBI patient to use.

Along with the technology, the various technologies are also available. TBI patients can use texting, emails, messaging services like WhatsApp and can send voice messages and make Wi-Fi calls. Communication in the post-modern world is a question of choice and option rather than a problem that needs to be solved.

MEMORY TOOLS

Impaired memory remains a problem for patients suffering from TBI. Various mechanisms and techniques are available and have been employed to help alleviate this problem.

Patients can start off with memory enhancement techniques. Conventional strategies for enhancement or improvement of memory include taking a mental snapshot, that is to say, visualize what needs to be remembered, albeit a phone number or time of an appointment. Exaggerate the image, add colors and sounds, distort the size and imagine bells and whistles, and experts and your memory will be significantly enhanced. Repetition, paying attention for longer than eight seconds and split information into units that can be remembered by sound and rhythm and every other form of enhancement, are all well-known methods. Other methods include cues, word associations, rhymes and acronyms

To compensate for impaired memory, it is helpful to write everything down and to place your notes in the same spot where it has always been visible to you and where you will develop the habit of looking to see the notes meant to remind you. Mobile phones contain every imaginable tool to aid memory, from note making systems to calendar and reminder systems and aids.

Keeping a journal and using black & whiteboards are also useful for keeping track of what should not be forgotten. One of the most underrated systems is to develop specific, consistent places to store important items. Always store your keys in a specific place and always place them there. The same goes for important papers, your mobile phone, glasses, and medicines.

Typical memory tools include calendars, personal organizers, mobile phone organizers, copiers, scanners, digital cameras, voice recorders, labeling machines, and phone recorders.

And, lastly, the old-fashioned way remains requesting reliable caregivers and friends to phone you, remind you and remember for you.

MOVEMENT & MOBILITY

Patients with TBI often experience impaired movement and mobility. This must be addressed and compensated for, and this begins with accepting the impairment's existence and allowing the patient more time to walk and move around and allow the patient much more time to prepare and get ready when he has to go to activities and appointments. What seems easy or fast for the unimpaired can be a very long process for the impaired. Transportation also has to be planned to accommodate the patient, to allow access and every form of transport has to be evaluated to assess suitability.

If the patient suffers from impaired walking or balance problems, she might be limited to certain activities and excluded from specific actions and activities. Some patients will not be able to climb ladders, walk down slopes or risk going onto slippery surfaces. If the patient's environment is planned according to his movement or mobility impairments, things can be organized around his ability to access by placing items within a closer range where he can reach for them easily. Physical therapy and proper assessment of her needs will go a long way towards improving their mobile quality of life.

Lack of movement, or impaired movement, can also have dangerous consequences. When someone does not move at all, the danger of blood clots becomes a real risk factor. Sequential compression stockings might be a wise addition to the equipment needs of the TBI patient to prevent clots from forming.

BEHAVIOR MODIFICATION

TBI patients can suffer from a great many mood and behavioral impairments. Often this becomes apparent quite simply when the

TBI patient seems to become passive and seems to lose interest in things they used to have a real passion for. The TBI patient might start to neglect hygiene and stop brushing their teeth unless someone reminded them to. Psychologists describe this as decreased initiation. Patients know what has to be done but are unable to get started with it. They might sit all day just staring into the distance, and even if someone prompts them to initiate some social activities to alleviate the lackluster sense of inaction, he will probably not get started with it anyway.

Lack of awareness, discussed above, has an obvious behavioral impact, and needs treatment and therapy not only to adapt but to alleviate symptoms and manage the environment too.

Another behavioral problem that requires modification is increased impulsivity. Psychologists often describe this in terms of the inability to inhibit certain behaviors rather than impulsivity. A damaged neural system, the inhibitor of behavior that causes the second reflection in our thinking - that allows for a pause to reconsider any actions before we actually do stuff – is often caused by damage to the prefrontal cortex. Patients suffering the same will sometimes come out with inappropriate statements (see more just below), do things that are literally ill-considered, and their actions will often be driven by instant gratification without any sense of insight in the probable ramifications. Impulsive spending and dangerous disregard for personal safety can be very perilous to these individuals.

In some of these patients, the disrupted behavior is embodied more by inappropriate or embarrassing social behavior rather than perilous impulsive behavior. Of course, a problem like this makes it very hard for the TBI patient to re-enter "society" or remain in the respective communities they belong to. It creates stigma and impacts family and caregivers more than perilous or dangerous behavior would.

Personal boundaries become vague, and the patients might start sharing intimate secrets with strangers or invade the private space of strangers by asking and discussing inappropriate private and personal matters in their lives. Oftentimes the patient will engage in inappropriate sexual gestures and behavior, or what might be considered vulgar discourse. For some, the use of foul language and constant swearing in inappropriate situations can become very problematic and even criminal.

The most common mood "disorder" that affect TBI patients is – as mentioned already, depression. Since depression and TBI injuries often intersect with symptoms like tiredness and lack of interest in life, the diagnosis, and treatment of depression in TBI patients is more complicated and need a higher level of training in the field of psychology/psychiatry as well as brain injuries in order to distinguish concomitant effects of brain injuries from the symptoms of depressive mood disorder.

Apart from depression, TBI patients suffer from post-traumatic stress disorder in many cases, resultant on the trauma of their accident and injuries. Anxiety is also a problem frequently reported. Changes in personal circumstances, the drain of resources and the impact on family life adds to this. Panic disorder is especially prevalent. All of these conditions have both neuropathological and psychosocial causes, and treatment can be complicated.

Apart from the above, anger and irritability – often embodied by quick-tempered outbursts or express irritability, some patients (infrequently reported) tend towards violence and aggression, although this is, fortunately, a rare manifestation. For some patients, it is emotions that become hard to control and not temper. These patients lose their emotional stability, and it seems as if they show a sort of bipolarity with emotions often exhibiting liability that disrupts their sense of contentment and inner peace. Some of these unfortunate patients may literally laugh themselves into tears of sadness, become sad and tearful when they come across scenes that would normally not have made an emotional impact on them, and laughter can to some extent, be disconnected with joy or humor and manifest in the most inappropriate situations when tears or visible displays of empathy might be more appropriate.

The aim of psychotherapy and especially, of caregiver and family support, is not in the first instance to cure the patient of these symptoms or mental ailments. The aim in the first place is to accommodate the behavior by understanding it and incorporating it into the total management of the care of the patient. Over time, some of the underlying causes of the behavioral problems might disappear as injuries heal, and the brain adapts, and sometimes therapy succeeds in developing compensatory strategies to keep the disruptive elements of the behavior in check. Sometimes, over long periods of time, the ailments can be cured by therapy.

RELEARNING SKILLS

A lot has been said about the relearning of skills above under the section about occupational therapy. Occupational therapy is often supported in this task by cognitive therapy that focuses on relearning many of the skills we lost and developing strategies and tools to compensate for abilities that might be lost forever. Some patients, though they did not lose the ability to read, lack the concentration to retain anything they read. These patients cannot read or talk without maintaining a state of hyper-vigilance which is tiresome and cannot be attained when they are not exceptionally well rested. For these patients, management of mental fatigue, including frequent naps and extended periods of rest after reading or writing, seems to retrain the brain, or at least, their mental fitness. The use of highlighters when reading for retention does seem to aid these patients' levels of concentration and makes continuity easier because the highlights leave a spore that can be traced back if they lose track. Reading as such improves the memory and redevelops the ability to concentrate, organize information and to retrieve information, so it is therapeutic as such. If the ability to read or write is completely lost, intensive occupational therapy will be required, and if needed, augmentation will be provided in the form of equipment and technology. This is a long process, and instant results are very unlikely.

When the receptive function of communication (listening or reading) or the expressive function (talking or writing) is impaired the TBI patient suffer from what can be described as hesitation in their speech when they are searching for a word or trying to keep on track with what they were trying to say. Similarly, the meaning of what we are being told is lost through misunderstanding and loss of concentration or even memory loss over the short term which deletes their recall of what the conversation is all about.

Some report that the use of email can help them overcome these problems, since they can, at any time, revert to the beginning, earlier conversations and they can spend more time in organizing their thoughts and narrative and search for the right words to express their point of view. Speech therapy might be required by patients who suffer the same. Various programs and aids for these patients are available on the internet.

CARETAKER FATIGUE

Severe TBI impacts the family and caregivers forever. Researchers report that high levels of emotional distress are reported even fifteen years after injury. And relationships amongst family members are affected and change negatively very often. Up to 45% of caregivers develop clinical levels of anxiety following the injury, while up to 47% of all caregivers develop depressive disorders.

As for the patient, the life of the caregiver family is forever changed after the injury. While all the effort is normally focused on the well-being of the patient, no service to support the caregivers exists. Isolation may cause the caregivers to end up in a bubble, believing that they are alone in their experience of stress and anxiety to cope with their task. As the levels of anxiety and stress, and plain old-fashioned fatigue, take its toll on the caregivers, their ability to support the patient is impaired, and this increases the pressure on the family. A vicious circle might develop and has to be taken care of by intervention if required. Sometimes something as simple as a bit of education accompanied by some reading materials will alleviate a lot of the caretaker anguish. If the family can develop stress management techniques, counseling and therapy, and practical support with problems like transport, things can quickly improve. It is regrettably, up to the caregiver to become aware of the deteriorating situation and they have to go look for or ask for support in most situations. Working with a social worker might benefit the family and bring a lot of support otherwise absent, to the household.

Typical stressors for the caregiver family include the annihilation of any self-time. Relaxation and enjoyment of the small things in life tend to be absorbed by feelings of guilt for what the injured patient might be missing in life, or simply become extinct due to the enormous task ahead of the family to take care of the needs of the TBI. Exhaustion can take over, and fatigue might become a constant companion. In the meantime, the financial strain is often very distressing. Not only does the income the patient might have brought in, disrupted, but the medical and rehabilitation costs, as well as the cost of equipment, transport, and medication, are often debilitating for a family budget.

Suddenly the husband may have to care for the children while being the caretaker and breadwinner, and sometimes the wife might have to become the breadwinner despite being responsible for the children and the household. Taking on both roles can be devastating to even the strongest amongst us.

Communication amongst family members and between caregivers and the patient is often severely disrupted. While the family members will often be completely unable to express their feelings about the situation, communication with the patient becomes impaired by the injury as well as by the repressed emotions of the caregivers who want to be there for the patient. Family events often become family meetings devoid of any social elements. Friends and other family members are often inclined to move away and to distance themselves from the caregiving family partly to escape the trauma they experience, and partly to remain uninvolved from any sense of duty to participate in responsibilities of care. Friendships may wither away, and the social life of the family might become a thing of the past.

All these elements and potential problems, and the caregivers' awareness of the potentiality of these detrimental aspects can lead to a total loss of the self and absorption in the caregiving role. Fatigue, loneliness, isolation, depression, and frustration might result to the detriment of all.

It is of the utmost importance that the caregiving family approach the task ahead of them with direct awareness of the potential caregiver burnout and that strategies and support systems and scheduled prevention of the loss of the self are planned and managed from day one. It is crucial to open up and allow social workers, friends and family access to the world of the caregivers and that mutual support and counselors and even psychotherapists are invited in. Joining support groups offer the best inoculation against caregiver burnout and can even change the injury and caregiving experience into a positive experience that brings the family and community closer together. Irrespective of one's views on this, prevention of caregiver fatigue has to be a number one priority for any family that wants to survive and flourish in the long run.

CHAPTER 4

Long-term goals

WHY TBI OUTCOMES ARE DIFFERENT FOR EVERY PATIENT

The long-term impact of TBI is notoriously difficult to predict. One of the main reasons for this is the fact that every TBI is unique. The amount of force, the direction of the force, location of impact, the health and the strength of the patient, the speed and quality of the treatment of the injury, all these factors determine the severity of the long-term effects of a TBI to some degree.

Recent research[v] elucidated how the individual patient's immune system and microbiota impact the severity of the TBI. Disruptions of the gut-brain axis appear to be partly responsible for ongoing TBI complications, and some suggested immune system treatment targets might improve future outcomes. The role of inflammation caused by the TBI is also under the microscope.

At best, predicting the outcome is a very complex and unchartered field in brain medicine. Because of the side effects caused by head injury, including some of the above-mentioned reactions inside the body, there might be a slight deterioration in the condition of brain cells over time, which may cause new symptoms or cause some of the long-term effects of TBI to become more severe.

According to McMillan, et al[vi] evidence is accumulating that TBI might trigger a persistent chronic disease with late deterioration - sometimes several years after injury. Studies show that up to 25% of all TBI survivors show functional deterioration between seven and thirteen years after injury, which might indicate that TBI could be the substrate for the induction of chronic: neurodegenerative processes.

Studies show that individuals who had a history of sick-leave or unemployment before their TBI suffered worse outcomes and had more problems with daily activities over the long-term than those fully employed with no history of frequent sick-leave. Studies also indicate that the longer the delay before discharge from intensive care and admission to rehabilitation, the worse the outcome was for the patient one year after injury.[vii]

The Angi Rubino Story

Angi was 14 years old when it happened. She was asleep in the back of her parents car when the impact to her head caved in the back half of her skull. She was in a coma for more than a month after undergoing a brain operation that lasted 18 hours.

It took her a year to relearn basic skills, like eating, walking and talking, and then she managed to go back to school.

Although her speech remained slow and nasal, few people noticed the change in her if they did not know her before her injuries.

Angi overcompensated for her injuries by working three times harder than anybody else. She became a classic over-achiever in life, but even her almost super-human effort and sterling college achievement could not ensure the career success she worked for.

The outcome for Angi in the end, was huge student debt and an inability to take care of herself. In retrospect, Angi feels that she should have taken things a bit easier. By overcompensating for her injuries, she set unrealistic goals for her future.

There is a consensus that the neuropsychiatric & functional sequelae (conditions resulting from a previous injury) are very amenable to treatment. Some of the determinants are:

The Michael Parks Story

Michael was hurt when the high pressure machine he was working on exploded and he was hit on the right side of his head by a broken. The blast blew him over a ledge and he fell six feet, hitting the concrete floor head first.

Mike was in a coma for more than a month. He woke up with absolutely no memory of the accident. He lost all his teeth and suffered from severe brain swelling. He was confused and had no idea who he was, where he was or how he got there. He was hospitalized for nine months before he was discharged to go home.

Several months after his discharge from hospital Mike's problems started. It began with seizures and migraines and he developed a severe depression. His memory deteriorated and he experienced constant pain. Years later, he still suffers from constant pain, and his memory is unreliable. Some days he has to use Google Maps to find his way home.

Early-stage involvement in neuro-rehabilitation is proven to improve long-term outcome. Even early education of both the family and the patient, accompanied by psychosocial support, improves long-term outcome. Rational pharmacotherapy – the administration of pharmacological treatment (drugs) that are evidence-based (treatments that have been scientifically proven to treat TBI) and based on the neuroanatomy and neurochemistry of the patient (his injuries), has been proven to improve acute and long-term disability following TBI.

VOCATIONAL TRAINING AND OCCUPATIONAL THERAPY

To live is to work. Having a job is the key to independence and social integration. And after a TBI, a so-called return to work plan (RTW) requires strong intervention and continued support from various people and institutions.

THE STEVE SMART STORY

Steve fell onto concrete, hitting the back of his head. He spent ten days in ICU and has absolutely no recollection of the first seven days afterward.. According to his family he was wide awake during this period and recognized everyone that came to visit.

For the first three weeks after being discharged home, he felt constantly dizzy but the dizziness disappeared after he was fitted with a neck brace.

After some time, he noticed that his personality was changing. He felt as if he was becoming someone else. Over time, his friends stopped calling. Steve describes watching himself go crazy and being unable to do anything about it. He was fired from his job because of his constant aggressiveness.

His wife stuck it out, and over time Steve learned to gain some control over his anger and established a somewhat altered identity. He remains distrustful and after three years his severe headaches are fading away and becoming much less severe. He remains somewhat ter and slightly dysthymic.

As with all caregiving and rehabilitation of TBI patients, nothing can be accomplished outside of a team effort, and the same goes for RTW.

The RTW team might include physiatrists (a medical doctor specializing in Physical Medicine and Rehabilitation), job coaches, social workers, physical therapists, occupational therapists, vision therapists, speech therapists, and neuropsychologists. Of course, nothing can happen, even when all these specialists are included, if the family and caregivers are not on board too.

The grand aim of this intervention is to assist the patient with all the requirements that have to be met in order to find a job and to develop the necessary compensatory skills to function well at work. Assistance is provided for job-placement and limited intervention afterward. What is called supported employment, which includes individualized support by a vocational rehabilitation specialist/job coach, has a job retention rate of over 70%.

The search and placement for the severe TBI patient becomes a process. After supporting the TBI patient up to the level where she is hired, the coach stays involved by facilitating both on-and off-site supports for the patient.

The coach remains involved, supporting the patient by developing strategies for her to succeed in reaching the skill levels required by the employer. The coach remains in the background and is available for assistance when new challenges arise, or new skills are required.

Another definition for an occupational therapist is someone who is trained to enable people to participate in everyday life by enhancing their abilities and/or modifying their environment to better support participation.[viii]

The activities of daily life that interest occupational therapists are normally divided into self-care, instrumental tasks (interacting with the environment) and complex tasks (like using public transport or managing personal finances).

Where the vocational coach intervenes specifically in order to facilitate the RTW plan, the occupational therapist has a wider field of intervention. The occupational therapist (OT) is not only involved in physical fitness, but also in the emotional and social adjustment of the patient into a larger society.

The OT is involved starting off with the acute care of TBI, to the return of the patient to normal life as a member of civilized society.

OTs will approach their task by developing exercises and activities that can simulate those needed by the TBI patient in order to adjust. By taking part in real life activities repetitively, patients can relearn movements they had lost due to their injuries.

Their task also includes the education of the caregivers, family members and their patients about procedures, safety, and the impairments that patient suffers from. Apart from this educational task, the OT is also involved in the process whereby the home of the TBI patient is modified to facilitate the patient's impairments, as well as an assessment of the patient's workplace environment, its accessibility and safety for the patient. In this role, she is a member of the RTW team.

It is important to note that one of the aims of occupational therapy[ix] is the quality of life of the patient. One of the determinants of a patient's quality of life is his ability to take part in meaningful occupations. Often, satisfaction in life as a whole correlates with the successful return to work, although some studies suggest that no such correlation exists for TBI patients because the TBI patient's work situation changes markedly.

IMPACT ON RELATIONSHIPS

Pondering questions of identity and change is as old as Western philosophy itself. Aristotle already pondered the issue deeply 24 centuries ago with the ship of Theseus thought experiment.

He wondered - if the Theseus, a famous wooden warship, was towed into the harbor as a museum piece, surely some of the wooden planks and parts would rot and perish as time went by, so the museum keepers would replace and restore all the rotten wood over the years. After a century or more, every single piece of wood of the original Theseus will be replaced. None of the original planks would remain. Aristotle wondered whether this restored wooden ship, ????

Patients who suffered TBI often change, emotionally, physically and temperamentally. For loved ones, the behavioral changes that they observe can be very distressing. For some, it is hard to accept that the injured person is actually the same person. It was Aristotle wondered whether the restored ship was still the Theseus, or was it an entirely different ship was still the same "object" as the original – or was it an entirely different vessel?

Twenty-four centuries later the family members and loved ones of TBI patients face the same problem. When the TBI patient is discharged and returns home, his injuries are marked, and nothing highlights the harm suffered more than the perceptible changes in the patient's behavior and emotional persona. Since more men than women suffer TBI, it is often the loving wife who is confronted with a changed man. Her husband might have been a sensitive and demonstrative lover and partner before his accident, and now her husband seems like a stranger to her. He might have changed into a selfish and garish lout who becomes agitated if his inappropriate sexual assertions are rejected by repulsed strangers.

The women (and men) in this *Theseus* moment in their lives, cannot be blamed if they become deeply thoughtful and struggle with the question: Is he the same man I married/loved? Or is he someone else now?

In one Guidebook for Psychologists, a spouse is quoted: *"We have two children, but **now I feel like I have three**."* Almost one in three women in this situation reportedly suffers verbal abuse, and more than 50% felt that although they were married, they did not have a husband, while 30% confided that they were for all practical purposes married to a stranger.

Every aspect of TBI stacks the deck against the patient when it comes to personal relationships. Many patients experience language problems, and since language, the ability to express and interpret emotions and to conceptualize the appropriate response in words, is essential for maintaining relationships, many patients start off with an inability to form a new relationship and real difficulty in maintaining existing ones.

Emotionally, many TBI patients remain vulnerable, and they often cannot deal with normal family and relationship issues. Impaired social skills make relationships inexplicable to those who cannot do or say the socially expected things we need to, in order to fit in and get along with others, and the ability to read people and situations are often impeded.

The emotional and physical closeness and sexual intimacy can be severely disrupted after TBI. The patient may experience diminished sexual interest or changing interests and activities.

Children often have a hard time too. They worry about their hurt parent's pain and suffering, but they also quickly pick up on strain and changes in the relationship of their parents, and these feelings are often internalized.

The children may become moody and withdrawn, lose interest in schoolwork and develop depression. Often, the children will experience some forms of guilt or self-doubt, and this may inhibit their youthful exuberance and rob them of their childhood. It is important to ensure that the children remain, children, whenever possible.

When children take part in the caregiving of a parent, supervision and careful consideration is very important. The caregiving experience is a reversal of the child-parent relationship and could be harmful to young children especially.

Communication with the children in caregiving households is the key to stability and continuance. Especially with older children who are going through puberty and into adolescence, great care should be taken not to appear patronizing or dishonest. Parents in this position should be patient and give them ample time to speak their minds. Listen to them and give them the facts. Make sure the teens, and all the children, understand that the changes they see in their parent are caused by the injuries to the brain.

In a post-modern cyber-world, the language of computing might actually make more sense to young people than medical explanations. *An injured brain, compared to a computer with bad sections that refuses to boot up properly resulting in a lower megahertz range and impaired ram memory,* might make more sense to modern teens than explanations that describe a traumatic injury to the occipital lobes, for example.

Of course, it is not only the immediate family that is affected by the TBI. The parents of the patient might feel that they should be more involved in the treatment and care for their son or daughter. They might even disagree vehemently sometimes, with the decisions made for care and rehabilitation, and they might resent not being in charge of looking after their beloved and injured child.

No one in the family can escape the distress and disruption. Everyone will have a point of view on what is best, based on their individual relationship with the patient. If family relations were strained before the accident, this would more often make matters worse afterward.

The only solution to these kinds of typical family issues is to involve as many members of the family as possible, to really consult everyone respectfully, by actually considering all advice and trying to incorporate as many good ideas as possible. Developing adequate "advocacy" skills to represent your beloved's interest is just another piece of the struggle for caregiver-spouses.

PSYCHOLOGICAL HEALTH

Patients who suffer from TBI often suffer tremendously. Research indicates that suicide is up to four times more likely amongst TBI survivors than amongst members of the general population *with major depression and no history of TBI.*

Substance abuse, hostility, and aggression are the strongest predictors of suicide amongst TBI patients. And shockingly, TBI patients who develop mood disorders and substance abuse after their injury are 21 times more likely to commit suicide than any non-TBI patient.

Research shows that substance use and abuse declines in the period shortly after a TBI, but over the long-term, substance use shows a marked increase. Studies have shown that up to 20% of abstainers and light drinkers become heavy drinkers after their TBI.

For patients of TBI, alcohol use is perilous, the more severe the injury, the more dangerous it can be. Not only can the use of alcohol have an amplified effect on the cognition and judgment of TBI patients, it actually correlates with significant morbidity.

Abstinence is the intelligent choice for TBI patients. Apart from the above-mentioned risks, alcohol sometimes becomes a trigger for seizures in the TBI patient. Seizures can be dangerous and is a horrid experience for patients and caregivers.

The use of alcohol and other substances should be discussed, and caregivers and the patient have to delineate guidelines that the patient has to adhere to. Counseling about the risks and side-effects has to be provided to the patient and the family, and no alcohol should be consumed before consultation with the medical practitioners involved in the treatment and care of the patient.

Alcohol can delay the healing process of the patient's brain. It will further impair the patient's thinking, react negatively with medications, make inappropriate behavior more likely, disable the patient's sense of balance even more severely, promote more risky behavior, and as mentioned above, increase the risk of seizures. None of these effects will offer anything positive for the TBI patient drinker.

In some cases, the only way to control or prevent self-harming substance abuse by the patient is to remove any form of alcohol or drugs from the home and to prevent the patient from somehow ordering more for home delivery.

Depression is one of the most prevalent side effects of TBI. In some patients, symptoms caused by the brain injury, itself, may simulate the symptoms of depression (low activity levels, difficulty controlling emotions), and expert intervention is required to diagnose major depressive disorder as a distinct condition. However, a great [percentage of TBI patients develop depression after their injury.

Caregivers must be on the lookout for signs of depression. Sometimes these symptoms are subtle. Male patients often report fatigue and irritability, sleep disturbances and a lack of interest in pleasurable activities when they are depressed.

Women will most likely report sadness, anxiety, feelings of guilt or increased appetite when they become depressed.

If the TBI patient suddenly becomes vivid and hurried to make a will or get their "things in order" or start distributing possessions amongst friends and family members, it might be time to start worrying. If they suddenly seem to feel surprisingly upbeat and talks about buying a gun or begin to stockpile medications, the patient might be very suicidal.

Caregivers can only offer emotional support and understanding. Patience and empathy in confronting the patient's depression can help. When talking with the patient, listen carefully, remain deeply thoughtful and do not diminish the patient's thoughts or feelings. Acknowledge the significance of his experiences and emotions, and carefully point out some alternate realities and rays of hope. It is very important to attempt to get the patient involved in as many activities as possible. Activity kills depression, just as depression kills activities, albeit it church services, shopping, movies or family gatherings. While these interventions are important, they should be subtle, and nothing should be forced upon the injured loved one. Get help.

TBI patients suffer from anxiety, and it is reported that the treatment of full-blown anxiety disorders are even more difficult to treat in TBI patients than treating depression or substance abuse.

Some anxiety is perfectly normal. Fears over diminished capacity are understandable. The patient cannot do everything they used to do, might fear social contact, permanent brain damage, losing his/her job and not being able to take care of their own physical needs.

Therapists report that improved problem-solving skills often help TBI patients to reduce stress and anxiety. When occupational therapists or psychotherapists teach patients how to solve problems, and systematic approaches to problem-solving, the TBI patients feel empowered, and some of their fears dissipate.

While the treatment of full-blown anxiety or panic disorders falls in the domain of professional medical intervention, family members and caregivers can play an important role in helping the patient relax and manage their fears and anxiety.

Engage the patient to understand what they do and partner with them to try to find a possible solution for their problems. Try to persuade the patient to start a journal to write down their fears and worries. Experience has shown that organizing your thoughts in this way can ease anxiety and slow down the anxious mindset.

If all else fails, it will help if the loved one can subtly change the topic or focus the patient's mind on something else – to distract the patient from his anxiety for a while.

If required, the caregiver can suggest that the patient speaks to his doctor about possible medication and counseling for his condition. Therapy might teach the patient various coping techniques that might reduce his levels of anxiety.

RECOVERY AND HEALTH, HOPE AND PEACE

Reinhold Niebuhr's famous serenity prayer still says it all.

> "God, grant me the serenity to accept
> the things I cannot change,
> Courage to change the things I can,
> And wisdom to know the difference."

The key to long-term functionality (mentally, physically and emotionally) for TBI patients and caregivers begins and ends with acceptance, courage, and wisdom – traits that result from endurance and perseverance.

In an ironic twist of fate, happiness and long life for TBI patients depend on the very same determinants that provide happiness and longevity to caregivers and uninjured people.

Employment and education provide the space for the cultivation of a healthy lifestyle and enjoyment of life and leisure. If the lifestyle is healthy, and contributes to physical, cognitive and emotional health and well-being, and, for the patient, to optimal recovery, peace of mind and optimism for the future will follow. And this is the essence of a good life.

Getting there is a bit more difficult for the TBI patient and his family and caregivers. Life interrupted, poses a bigger challenge and demands more and harder efforts to overcome on the way to the Promised Land.

The brain remains a mysterious and most complex organ. Science still cannot fully explain how the brain heals after injury, or what exactly goes on during the recovery from TBI. Opinions differ.

One school of thought believes that the remaining healthy brain tissue somehow takes over from damaged brain tissue and slowly learns how to do what the damaged brain used to do.

Another school of thought posits that brain recovery is all about the rearrangement of neurons and the reconnection of brain cells that naturally tends towards efficiency.

What we do know is that the brain can, in fact, heal itself to some degree. Younger brains recover faster and easier than older brains. Obviously, more severe injuries take longer and remain more damaged than light injuries, and the location of the injuries play a big role in determining the outcome.

Interestingly enough, the recovery of the injuries to the brain is partly determined by the totality of the injuries the patient sustained all over his body. The more severe the body is damaged – fractures, bleeding, trauma and organ damage, etc. – the longer the brain will most likely take to recover. It is almost as if the body has a limited power supply and the more injuries, the less power available for the brain itself to take care of itself.

In the same way, the healthier the body is, and the healthier the lifestyle the TBI patient follows, the more energy and healing power the brain will be able to tap into. A life free from addiction, mental illness, obesity, and inactivity, will produce a body that can spend much more effort on healing the brain.

The health of the body is often uniquely connected to sleep patterns. Healthy sleeping habits optimize health and recovery, but sleeping patterns for TBI patients are easily disrupted and need constant monitoring.

TBI patients often develop insomnia and wake up frequently during the night. Because they often remain awake at night, excessive daytime sleepiness might drive them to overly frequent daytime napping, which can further disrupt their sleep hygiene.

It is often advised that TBI patients should endeavor to limit their daytime naps. This should be done after consultation with medical practitioners. Many strategies and methods exist to ensure healthy sleeping.

Avoidance of coffee and soda after lunch, exercise, having an early supper, regular and fixed bedtimes and rising times, a quiet and dark bedroom and not spending any time in bed or doing anything in bed apart from sleeping, all contribute to a disciplined and healthy sleeping cycle.

Sleep health is not only a co-determinant of bodily health but especially of emotional health too. Physical and emotional health remains interconnected with disturbances in one leading to impairments in the other.

Diet and exercise are two further determinants of health. While the body of a TBI patient may become more passive – or inactive – the appetite of the individual might remain based on previous activity levels. The intake of TBI patients has to be carefully monitored. Obesity, already a very limiting condition for uninjured individuals, can become a severely disruptive force in the life of a TBI patient.

The health of caregivers strangely impacts the health of the patient. When the caregiver develops what is popularly known as caregiver fatigue, or compassion fatigue, despair often becomes a real presence in their lives. Despair borne from frustration, feelings of being trapped, fear that the patient is not recovering as fast and as completely as everyone expected and hoped for, and despair borne out of pure old-fashioned fatigue.

A caregiver burnout displaces elements to the patient, who will feel some sense of hostility or develop guilt, or who may simply have difficulty understanding his sense of negativity, which he/she might turn on themselves.

To prevent this from happening caregivers have to look after themselves first. They have to carefully monitor their own diet, exercise, leisure, and recreation, alcohol use and mood swings, hope, and optimism. It is essential for caregivers to find a positive outlet where they can recharge and recoup their sense of self on a regular basis if they want to keep up with the demands of caregiving and the effect their wellness has on the patient.

In order to relieve the tension and get rid of any toxic feelings, someone to talk to is absolutely non-negotiable. Significant others or family members that care, support groups or even therapy, can make a world of difference. Anyone with whom the caregiver can talk without being judged or offered ill-advised opinions will do the trick. Sometimes medications might be required to keep on track. Needless to say, tobacco use should be avoided, and alcohol and drug use limited.

Some families are more naturally inclined to conform, and maybe to find peace and acceptance when they cannot change their fate. Some families tend to be more existential, and sometimes these families vent their unwillingness to just accept what they cannot change – now – with the feverish pursuit of technological breakthroughs and alternative cures.

Time is often the great healer. Human beings learn to accept their fate over time, and as time goes by, we all have the capacity to adapt and find happiness irrespective of our lot. The same goes for the majority of TBI patients. When the body is injured and the mind disrupted, our experience of illness changes our perspective of life to some extent. This is nature's way to make life bearable.

With time and support – with loving care, attention and healthy optimism, most people learn to accept their fate, to find meaning in their suffering, and to make peace with their limitations rather than focusing on their remaining gifts and abilities. Spiritual counseling can play an important role for many people during the journey.

Once patients and caregivers, and everyone else for that matter, succeeds in finding their own voice, a voice apart from mental illness, brain injury, regrets and guilt, pain and suffering, they realize sooner or later that this is their one life. When this is truly understood, peace is more often than not the result.

CHAPTER 05

Mild TBI and concussion

Mild TBI, or concussion, is delineated from severe TBI in the first instance by the loss of consciousness. In short, mild TBI can be defined as an injury that may cause the loss of consciousness for 15 minutes or less, or according to the World Health Organization's definition, a loss of consciousness for 30 minutes or less.

Memory loss for events just before or after the incident might present, and the patient will most likely feel confused and bewildered. Mild TBI can be a very misleading diagnosis. A very large percentage of brain injuries start off with a "mild" diagnosis and end up with quite severe complications, so care has to be taken not to misunderstand the dangers inherent in so-called mild brain injuries.

Some medical practitioners designate slightly more severe *"mild"* injuries as moderate traumatic brain injuries. Patients, who lose consciousness between fifteen minutes and a few hours, can be diagnosed as moderate. According to theory, symptoms of moderate TBI fall somewhere between mild and severe TBIs.

IMPACT

Approximately 50% of patients with mild traumatic brain injuries (MTBI) suffer some symptoms. Physically, the patients can experience blurred vision, dizziness, and fatigue, headaches, nausea and sleep disruption.

Anxiety is a frequent problem. Many patients suffer from confusion and bewilderment, and depression is almost ubiquitous. To accompany these symptoms, many patients report that they experience emotional lability and varying degrees of irritability.

MTBI also impacts the cognitive functioning of patients. Apart from confusion and bewilderment, many patients report impaired memory (especially short-term), decreased concentration and attention span, a sense of mental functioning slowing down.

Almost 85% of patients, according to research done in the UK, recover fully within one week after the MTBI, and up to 97% are symptom-free after one month. Of course, the quality and speed of recovery various and are co-determined by age and health prior to the injury.

To put these very positive reports into a bit more realistic perspective, it will take up to three months before 88% of these patients are able to go back to full-time work. In the USA studies reported that only approximately 73% of MTBI patients would eventually return to their previous jobs. Regrettably, approximately 5% of MTBI patients will experience ongoing symptoms.

There is as yet no consensus on the prevalence of ongoing disabilities after (apparently) mild TBI. A recent study in Scotland shocked the medical fraternity when it was reported that between 42% and 52% of patients who were hospitalized with MTBI suffer ongoing moderate or severe disabilities.

According to Stocchetti and Zanier[x] 50% of MTBI recovered complete cognitive competency, while only 20% required some assistance; the incidence of seizures in patients with MTBI & moderate TBI are between 5% and 10%.

The majority of these patients will suffer from impaired concentration, memory and organizing skills and some will find it severely difficult to focus on anything for sufficient periods of time, although many of these symptoms can resolve on their own over time.

The most important insight to be derived from studying MTBI is to understand that despite the fact that the injury might be less severe, it will be a huge mistake to equate the apparently less severe (injury) cause of symptoms with the real impact on the physical, cognitive and emotional functioning of the patient.

A subset of patients with MTBI will suffer persistent disability, and these patients will require specialized intervention. Various rehabilitation strategies for the treatment of these patients have been developed over time. As long as the patient has access to medical services and this is provided in time, management of the symptoms can alleviate a lot of the patient's suffering.

COPING WITH MTBI

One of the problems patients with MTBI face is a discrepancy between their own experience of the severity of their MTBI symptoms and the perceptions of their family members. Often the family members are unaware of the extent of the symptoms the patient suffers. This can be partly due to the fact that symptoms of MTBI are often more subtle and less visible to the family. The patient might be having real difficulties in thinking and can suffer severe distress without the family taking cognizance of his condition. As a consequence, the patient and the family might end up with widely divergent ideas about the goals for further treatment and rehabilitation.

This can be especially detrimental to the survivor of MTBI. The family support system is a crucial and irreplaceable part of the patient's rehabilitation and recovery and is instrumental in the planning of the patient's long-term care. For this reason, for MTBI, greater care should be taken to obtain multiple viewpoints about the patient's current functioning and goals. In this scenario, care has to be taken not only to ensure that that family members and caregivers have an understanding of the levels of awareness of the patient about her strengths and weaknesses, but inversely, also to double-check that caregivers and family members have a real understanding and awareness of the patient's real and perceived strengths and weaknesses.

Consensual wisdom in the treatment of MTBI exists in broad terms. In order to optimize the rate and quality of recovery, the patient has to rest and rest a lot. Resumption of pre-injury tasks, activities, and responsibilities has to be gradual and controlled. Hasty resumption of "normal" activities can be very harmful and counterproductive. Older patients and especially patients who have had previous brain injuries must take unusual care to take it slow and to be patient – being in a hurry can be especially harmful to these individuals.

For most patients who survive MTBI, complete recovery can be expected after three months. If symptoms persist after three months, this might indicate the persistence of symptoms requiring intervention and ongoing treatment and management.

To complicate matters even more for the patient with MTBI, some health practitioners classify MTBI into two distinct categories, namely uncomplicated MTBI (UMTBI) or complicated MTBI (CMTBI).

An injury is classified as UMTBI if no problems can be seen on a CT scan or MRI of the brain. An injury is classified as CMTBI if some abnormalities are observed on a CT scan or MRI of the brain. Abnormalities refer to bruising or the collection of blood in the brain. Patients with CMTBI can experience longer-term outcomes.

HEADACHES

Headaches are the most common somatic complaint for patients with MTBI. Prolonged headaches are very disruptive for family life, recreation, and employment. These headaches sometimes occur not because of the brain injury itself but because of injuries that occurred during the incident that impacted the rest of the body. When the headaches do originate from the brain injury itself, it is often due to neurochemical abnormalities, damage to nerve fibers or disrupted cerebral circulation. Headaches are expected, as a rule, to resolve within six to twelve months after the injury, but some patients suffer from headaches for much longer, some even permanently.

In 20% of cases, pain is caused by a trauma-triggered migraine. A trauma-triggered migraine is much more common in patients who have had a previous record or family record of migraines. For treatment of migraine headaches, a variety of drugs are prescribed, from Beta-blockers and calcium-channel blockers to antidepressants and antiepileptics.

Many patients also suffer from tension headaches. These headaches, also known as stress headaches or muscle contraction headaches, can last anything from 30 minutes to seven days always without presenting nausea or vomiting and characterized by non-throbbing. Medications prescribed for tension headaches include non-narcotic pain treatment, muscle relaxants, and anti-inflammatory drugs.

It takes time by trial-and-error to find the right medicine to treat headaches, and the patient should never digress from the doctor's precise instructions.

Fatigue and stress can exacerbate headaches in patients with MTBI, so taking care of these symptoms may help to relieve the pain suffered from headaches. There are other options for treatment of headaches. Sometimes physical conditioning of the neck through stretching and strengthening exercises can relieve symptoms. Healthcare practitioners sometimes instruct patients to swim in warm water. This can help to loosen the muscles which may bring relief. Alternative treatments like acupuncture and occipital nerve blocks are helpful. Some patients rely on physical therapy. Botox and biofeedback have also been reported to alleviate headaches.

Family members and caregivers can be helpful too. The MTBI patient can be persuaded to lie down in a dark and quiet room. Sleeping can alleviate symptoms, as mentioned above. Application of heat or ice can also be helpful, but it is advisable to first consult the patient's doctor before going application.

Light sensitivity can also be a cause. Avoidance of bright lights (sunlight) should be avoided and wearing sunglasses can be helpful. Avoidance of foods and beverages that are known to cause headaches (coffee, alcohol, chocolate) as a part of the overall strategy will do no harm either. Basic stress management will also go a long way in preventing headaches. Rest, relaxation and recreation can help to minimize the side-effects of stress.

SLEEP PATTERNS AND LIFE ROUTINE

Changes in sleep patterns are common for almost all patients who suffer from TBI. From the outset, patients should get as much sleep as possible during the night. Although it is important to rest during the day, long periods of sleep during the day should be avoided because it might lead to insomnia at night.

For those that suffer from sleep initiation problems, a variety of medications can be prescribed, including amitriptyline. Those suffering from sleep maintenance problems can be prescribed nortriptyline.

Research has shown that patients with MTBI need more sleep. Patients and caregivers need to take heed of this. If the MTBI patient attempts to sleep the same amount after the injury, constant fatigue and exacerbated memory problems will most likely become a problem.

The development of healthy sleeping patterns must be a shared responsibility that includes the participation of the health care team. It is paramount that the patient avoids caffeine. Limiting or completely avoiding tea, coffee and energy drinks, even soda, will help to restore healthy sleep patterns.

Exercise is a sleep aid, but not if the exercise is done close to bedtime. Build a routine where the patient has his last meal about four hours before bedtime and limit fluid intake two hours before. The core of a sleep pattern is a fixed routine. The patient should get up at the same time every morning, and ideally, should go to bed at a fixed time at night. Also, avoid "living" in bed. The bed should ideally only be used for sleep (or sex) and not for eating, watching television or reading.

A dark bedroom without distractions from flashing lights and electronic gadgets and mobile phone sounds and flashes will aid peaceful sleep. It is advised that the patient gets out of bed when she cannot sleep. Watching television and reading or any similar activity until she feels really tired again, will relieve her from the stress of waiting for sleep, trying to fall asleep, and focusing on being awake.

To aid the patient's ability to return to normal routine functionality, the family should assume the responsibility to implement a plan to establish a daily structure that includes consistent times for all activities. The whole family must understand the plan and the goal of the plan, and no plan can be implemented without the involvement of the patient and without giving the patient some choices and some control over his own life routines. To produce a workable structure and routine, the impairments of the patient must be taken into consideration, and compensatory strategies have to be implemented. The use of day planners, alarms, phones with large buttons and medicine dispensers, etc. should be relied upon.

A so-called master schedule is often recommended for caregivers. A master plan for every day of the week should be drawn up. It should structure life for the patient and the caregivers and help to re-establish a routine and life structure for the patient. A typical master plan should include time to wake up, breakfast and medication time, dressing and grooming, physical activity and rest, lunch and bathroom, therapy and dinner, leisure and recreation, and bedtime activities and time to go to sleep.

MOOD

MTBI patients often experience a variety of feelings and emotional changes. Depression is ubiquitous, and many patients experience mood swings and anxiety too.

When the MTBI patient becomes depressed, emotional support is the primary gift the caregiver and family members can offer. Being there, being supportive and showing understanding and patience will go a long way. Encouragement is important, and caregivers should avoid offering rash solutions and clichéd reactions to the MTBI patient's sense of hopelessness. The type of encouragement that is beneficial is one that underscores the real existence of depression but emphasizes the fact that the feeling of despair, like all things, will go away over time and that treatment will bring relief.

Often, all that is required is talking and listening actively. Offer hope, but not solutions. Just the acknowledgment of the patient's feelings is often enough to solicit a positive response. Depression is inactivity and involving the depressed patient in as many activities as possible, might already alleviate some of his feelings of depression.

Medical intervention might be required, and it is important not to wait for depression to heal itself before consulting the health care practitioner.

COGNITION

Cognition is dependent on thinking and memory skills. Healthy cognition is based on the ability to concentrate, to pay attention, to be aware of yourself, the environment and of other people – on having the ability to manage your affairs, to plan and organize your life, the ability to make decisions and implement plans, the ability to focus on problems and to come up with solutions, the soundness of mind to make realistic and appropriate judgments, all the while using reason and intellect.

Changes in cognition are very common for patients with MTBI. When the brain is injured, it is to be expected that thinking might be affected. Fortunately, the brain is unparalleled in its ability to heal, so many of the cognitive impairments that accompany MTBI improve and disappear over time, although cognitive healing often takes longer than physical healing.

Concentration problems are common. In practice, this means that the ability to focus the mind becomes impaired. This impairment comes in the form of distractibility. The more focused the mind becomes, the less aware we become of the environment. Someone who is concentrating 100% will probably not hear a gunshot in the next room. When the concentration is affected, patients will often not be able to concentrate when any distractions exist. Inability to follow a conversation in a cafeteria where there is a constant chatter all around, or the inability to listen to the radio for example, if the television is on with the sound turned down, would be typical examples. Reading pretty much requires total concentration, and this will be very hard to do if concentration becomes impaired.

Caregivers can support the patient who has difficulty concentrating by removing as many of the distractions as possible. Creating scheduled quiet times for the patient to focus his mind optimally and arranging the patient's bedroom or study/office to be calm, quiet and distraction-free will is a good start. For some patient's medication such as methylphenidate might be prescribed by a medical doctor, psychiatrist or neurologist.

One of the most important lifestyle determinants to enhance concentration, apart from diet and the introduction of supplements and foods like fatty acids and nuts, is to ensure that the patient never feels tired or fatigued, that sleep patterns are normal and healthy, that the patient sleeps at night and not mostly during the day, and that the patient is as relaxed and free from anxiety as possible. All the above disrupts concentration and impairs cognition.

Memory impairment is another very common cognitive problem suffered by many patients of MTBI. Patients, whose injuries impacted the anterior temporal lobes, will be especially affected by memory impairment. Short term memory is usually affected the most.

Forgetting names and dates, appointments and things (tools, phone, and keys) and the need to be repeatedly reminded, can be prevented and managed by using memory aids that might include written journals, diaries, lists, checklists and schedules, stick-it notes and alarms, even written explanation of events and situations that can be accessed when the memory just won't produce the required results.

The mind may also slow down significantly. This may slow the patient down, and as a result, the household. The patient might now take a very long time to answer questions, make choices or select from various options. Even movement might be slowed down as a result. Delayed reactions, even emotional slowness might occur, and the patient might take a very long time to grasp thing that she might have understood instantly before the injury.

Whether this slowdown is permanent or short-term, family members and caregivers must take care to compensate for the sake of the patient. Her frustration with her slowdown will often be much more severe than the family's frustration. Even more tragic - if the patient does not have any awareness of her slowdown, things could really become complicated. Patience and empathy are the only tools in the short term. Most likely these impairments will improve over time. If not, the family needs to develop more tools to compensate for them.

SEXUAL

It is often said in jest, that sexuality is all in the mind, but those who have witnessed loved ones suffer from TBI can often see the impact of even MTBI on sexuality. Sometime the only – shall one call it sexual impairment for lack of a better description – is a decreased sense of the appropriate. Patients who suffered MTBI sometimes lose their sense of propriety, and this can result in behavior which is frowned on in normal society. Inappropriate or even vulgar sexual gestures might be made towards age or gender inappropriate individuals or towards individuals with whom nonsexual relationship exist or can develop. Rude sexual comments and unwarranted sexual behaviors might cause discomfort and embarrassment for family members, strangers and the patient himself.

More often, however, patients experience changes and/or impairments in their sexuality, sexual functioning, and regulation of intimacy. Most common, are impairments that relate to levels of arousal, decreased libido and the inability to achieve orgasm. In rare cases, the opposite might happen, and the patient can suddenly become hypersexual. Erectile dysfunction and decreased sexual appetite are much more common though.

The injured partner often stops participating in foreplay and lose their interest in intercourse, sometimes due to severely reduced sexual self-esteem and a loss of sense of sex-appeal. Alienation forms the spouse often frequently reports. Changes in mood, depression, and medications often exacerbate these changes.

In rare cases, problematic sexual behavior might be very difficult for the family to manage. As mentioned, in very rare cases, hypersexuality might develop, and patients might lose their sense of civility by exposing themselves or masturbating in public. Promiscuity might become a problem, and sometimes obsessions with pornography and even aggressive attempts to engage in sex with strangers can become a real problem. Patients have been reported to even change their sexual orientation after injuring their limbic structure.

The above analysis should not be cause for extreme reaction. Many of the above-mentioned potentialities are so rare that it can almost be discounted, and many are even more unlikely to appear in the life of an MTBI patient. The main point is just to understand that sexuality and sexual functioning cannot escape from the effects of TBI.

Because of the intimate nature of sexuality, this is a topic that is often very hard to discuss or to expose to treatment, therapy, and medical practitioners. Therapists recommend that spouses and caregivers develop a way to signal the patient when he is saying something inappropriate. Sometimes it is possible just to change the subject before things go too far. Discussions with the injured family member about what is appropriate may help, and explaining that sexual feelings are normal but should remain private is recommended. The patient has to be given an outlet to express his sexual needs, so a private bedroom, for example, should be available.

The emotional and physical closeness a couple once enjoyed might be impaired after an MTBI. The medications used and the injury itself can lead to emotional withdrawal while the caregiving spouse might just be too tired and busy with her caregiving duties, in a sense, being a *mother* to the patient makes it hard to be a wife or lover too. For couples who do not have any children yet, the TBI can induce more stress and fear whether they would be able to conceive in the future.

Although time will often repair most of these impairments especially for the MTBI patient, counseling and therapy are highly advisable to help the couple navigate these difficult times without losing the magic that made their relationship work in the first place.

VOCATIONAL AND EDUCATIONAL EMPOWERMENT

We have discussed the role of vocational coaches and occupational therapists in some details above, so we will suffice with just a few remarks here.

Rehabilitation counselors specialize in providing personal and vocational counseling and training, and even job placement services, for their clients. Some state agencies also provide assistance. Vocational rehabilitation funding is available.

The job coach is available at the workspace to take care of the needs of the patient and will assist in developing compensatory strategies for the patient to be able to perform his task at the required level of compliance the employer demands.

Caregivers can support the patient if he is busy transitioning to a new job or if he decides to enroll for some training courses or even if he wants to continue with his studies or start studying in a new field. Support and assistance with scheduling and assistance in creating the most positive environment for the patient to start on a new journey such as this. It Is all that can be required from the family and all that the patient may need.

To accommodate MTBI patients who desire to go back to college, a lot can be done during the college selection phase to ensure the future student's success. According to the Individuals with Disabilities Education Improvement Act (IDEA, 2004) colleges are guided although not prescribed, to make access for disabled students equal and seamless.

Every college will adhere to the law in a different manner, so selecting the best option with the injuries of the MTBI in mind will take a bit of investigation. Assistive technology can make the world of difference to the student. AccessIT provides electronic and information technology specific for students with disabilities. The website contains millions of resources that can be searched for answers about electronic and information technology for the same.

DO-IT, another program (Disabilities, Opportunities, Internetworking and Technology) endeavors to increase the participation of disabled individuals in challenging academic programs and careers.

The sky is the limit for those individuals who are prepared to be pro-active despite their injuries.

PREVENTION AND RECURRENCE

The relative risk of recurrent TBI is measured to be at least 3.00 times higher than the risk of a first impact. Conversely, patients with MTBI (and severe TBI) who suffer from mild cognitive impairment may be at greater risk for recurrent TBI from fighting, falling or involvement in an accident, with increased risk for injury and delirium afterward.

Patients who suffer from MTBI who suffer recurrent MTBI have been indicated to have a very high risk of long-term neurocognitive impairment.[xi] Studies by Weiss et al. demonstrated that 25% of all brain injury survivors show deterioration in cognitive functions and earlier signs of aging. Of course, the more the cognitive functions deteriorate, the higher the risk of recurrent brain injury becomes.

Apart from the discussion above where preventative strategies were discussed relating to decluttering of the environment and some more, nothing is as important as building up strength and living as healthy as possible – and health starts with diet and nutrition. Neurotransmitters that help determine behavior and moods (dopamine, serotonin) are directly influenced by dietary intake. Foods that increase dopamine will make your mind clearer and more alert. Just so, ingesting foods that increase serotonin, will co-determine the improvement of anxiety levels.

If the body receives enough protein, injuries will heal faster and with less physical disruption. Enough of the right types of fats (like essential fatty acids) will support the body by strengthening the immune system, and this will assist the body in fighting inflammation that is partly responsible for the deterioration of brain injuries and the exacerbation of symptoms. If enough vegetables, especially green and cruciferous types are ingested, enough vitamins and minerals will be absorbed, and this will supply the body with all it requires to maintain the microbiota which co-determines the gut-brain connection that has been directly implicated in the recovery and prevention of inflammation of brain injuries, see above. Contrary to some writers, who advocate the need for large quantities of carbohydrates, research suggests that carbohydrates should be limited. The effect of ketones on epilepsy and other conditions are well documented.

Similarly, exercise, both aerobic and anaerobic (strength training) will improve the mental clarity and mood of the patient, but more importantly in this context, is the fact that fitness, strength, and endurance is a great preventative strategy not only to combat the possible fast-tracked aging path some MTBI patients can be exposed to, and the enhanced physical abilities will very importantly, reduce the likelihood of further TBI caused by falls, accidents, and reduced situational awareness.

Taking care is the most likely strategy to prevent further serious TBI and deterioration of brain health and symptoms. Taking care includes abstinence from tobacco, which is extraordinarily dangerous for MTBI patients, even more so than for the non-TBI population. Tobacco is harmful to the entire body and all its systems, but especially so for the brain. It is common knowledge that smoking *kills* brain cells, something that no one, especially no TBI patient can afford. By reducing oxygen intake, smoking also deprives the oxygen-hungry MTBI brain even more.

The same goes for alcohol and drugs, and inactivity poses almost the same risk as the aforementioned. Taking care is also especially focused on being very careful. In order to prevent further concussion and to minimize the risk of further head injuries, which would have catastrophic consequences for the MTBI patient, non-participation in any activities that can increase his risk should be a no-go. No touch football, no surfing, no motorcycle riding - and even cycling should either be avoided or done only while wearing a crisis quantity of protective gear. Avoidance of wet floors, tiles or the sidewalk after snow, ice or rain and wearing custom boots and slippers with rubber soles should be second nature. There is only one secret: prevention is better than cure.

SECTION C
LIVING YOUR BEST LIFE

CHAPTER 6

Additional Support

SUPPORT GROUPS

Support groups fulfill a very important function in the life after injury for virtually every survivor of TBI.

Members of these groups share strategies they developed to help them cope, and they feel a sense of belonging to a community of like-minded people.

Group members keep abreast with the newest developments and share information and understanding for each other's suffering.

These groups often provide a sympathetic environment where survivors can build social networks.

US BRAIN INJURY SUPPORT GROUPS

By visiting the THIS INDEX survivors and caregivers can access the website of the Brain Injury Peer Visitor Association. On this page, links are provided to websites for every State in the Union, and on these websites the details and locations for every Brain Injury Support Group in the United States is provided.

The journey from injury to TBI trauma recovery is a difficult one full of obstacles and discomfort for everyone involved, although it is not completely unrewarding and without joy.

Those who live with TBI, albeit patients or caregivers have many resources available thanks mainly, to the vastness of the modern internet. Support groups, social media forums, and raw databases are legion, but it is not so easy to find the best resource at the very moment when it's needed.

Leading websites managed by famous hospitals and rehabilitation facilities compete with private blogs and state & government pages to provide the public at large with all the information that exists on TBI. Digital resources include academic journals, publications and books of every conceivable nature on every conceivable aspect of traumatic brain injury.

This publication was conceived because of the vast network of information available. Although data on every aspect of TBI are available, there are very few, maybe no publications that gather all the relevant data and order it in the framework employed here meant to elucidate the journey from injury to life after TBI for the TBI patient and caregiving family.

APPENDIX ONE: SOME ONLINE RESOURCES

The Brain Injury Peer Visitor Association	A 501(c)(3) non-profit organization led by volunteers and dedicated to supporting TBI survivors and their families.	http://www.braininjurypeervisitor.org/index.php?p=1_3_About-Us
All in One Accessibility	A for-profit consulting firm that provides home modification/ renovations for survivors of traumatic injuries	http://www.allinoneaccess.com/
American Trauma Society	Dedicated to the elimination of needless death and disability from injury.	https://www.amtrauma.org/
Americans w. Disabilities Act	A link to all the relevant laws that might pertain to survivors of TBI	https://www.ada.gov/pubs/ada.htm
Brain & Life	The American Academy of Neurology's Magazine for survivors and caregivers interested in everyday living	https://www.brainandlife.org/
Brain Injury Association of America	To improve the quality of life of every person in the US affected by TBI.	https://www.biausa.org/
Caring Bridge	Offers free websites that support and connect members of the family and friends of patients in treatment and recovery.	https://www.caringbridge.org/
Caring for caregivers	Useful links & tips & stories for & about caregivers TBI survivors	http://www.braininjurypeervisitor.org/index.php?p=1_12_Caregivers
Help Hope Live	Fundraising site for medical expenses that the insurance will not cover	https://helphopelive.org/
Living with Brain Injury	LBI is an information center and a source of inspiration for TBI survivors, caregivers, family and friends	http://thebrainfairy.com/
Mobility Works	If you want to buy or rent a wheelchair accessible vehicle, this company has over 70 locations nationwide	https://www.mobilityworks.com/
Mortgage Loans	Mortgages and Home Loans for survivors of traumatic brain injuries	https://www.mortgageloan.com/disabilities

National Resource Center for Traumatic Brain Injury	The mission is to provide practical information for professionals, survivors and family members who struggle with TBI	http://www.tbinrc.com/
Return 2 Work	A 501(c)(3) Non-profit that organization that provides personalized vocational rehabilitation and employment services to Americans with disabilities	https://www.return2work.org/about-r2w/overview
Social Security Admin Work Site	For information you need when you want to work while on Social Security	https://www.ssa.gov/work/
Medicare Hotline	Financial assistance for survivors of TBI who are eligible	www.medicare.gov 800-633-4227

APPENDIX TWO: INJURY

DESCRIPTION	MILD TBI	SEVERE TBI
Duration Unconscious	Less than ½ hour	More than ½ hour – month or more
Bruising or Bleeding	None	Swelling, bruising or Bleeding
Duration of Amnesia	Brief, minutes to a few hours	Several days. Might last for months
Prognosis	Should recover fully within 3 months	Prime period of recovery within the first 12 months. Gradual improvements for the first two years
Impaired Cognition	Very few impairments after one year	Cognitive impairments are quite common after one year
Recovery Plan	Feedback from the injury survivor. The family may help to set goals. Keep limitations of the patient in mind.	Feedback from patient most likely unavailable or limited. Pair with goals set by family and must remain realistic
Realistic Recovery	Develop methods to compensate for impairments and gradual return to normal life.	Develop a new sense of self. Develop methods to cope with new levels of functionality
Persistent Impairments	Develop strategies to cope with persistent impairments. Focus on increasing functionality despite obstacles	First focus on the basic activities of daily life. Help to develop realistic life goals. Goals include resuming work or school. Emphasize community-based activities

APPENDIX THREE: DEALING WITH FATIGUE

Severe fatigue is one of the main problems a TBI survivor has to cope with. Strategies to manage fatigue are helpful
Use planning tools (calendar & alarms) to help the management of rest periods and naps on a regular basis. Try to limit naps to no more than ½ hour at a time during the morning and early afternoon
Do not resume activities faster than the management of fatigue allows
Start with simple tasks, and gradually attempt more tasks as fatigue becomes manageable
Be alert for the signs and symptoms of fatigue the patient might display. Sensitivity is a great fatigue management aid
During rehabilitation, breaks every 5 or 10 minutes is indicated to prevent fatigue
The use of a wheelchair & other aids during trips and visits might help prevent exhaustion
Carefully manage the energy sapped during visits and plan accordingly

APPENDIX FOUR: COGNITIVE IMPAIRMENT

IMPAIRMENT	SYMPTOMS	TIPS
Bewilderment	Becomes confused easily and has difficulty sticking to a schedule Has difficulty distinguishing timelines of events Invents explanations for events where a gap in memory exist	Use a notebook to record and list events and teach the patient to refer to his book during the day Develop a consistent routine for all tasks Do not randomly change routines Help the patient to fill in details where his memory lapses
Memory	Difficulty remembering any new short-term information Indicative if the patient cannot remember her schedule or program for any given day	Follow a fixed daily routine Write everything down in the working diary Repeat every relevant detail repeatedly during the day
Concentration	Easily distracted Simply cannot multi-task even the simplest activities Very short attention span	Never do more than one thing at a time Repeatedly check and regain the patient's attention Work in a quiet and closed environment Allow the patient to repeat as many of the mutual communication as possible
Decisiveness	The patient is making bad choices Cannot seem to solve problems Impaired reason Cannot make up his mind	Write options and pros and cons down in the diary Discuss the options in simple terms

IMPAIRMENT	SYMPTOMS	TIPS
Initiation	Despite best intentions, simply cannot get to it, and never does what she planned Lack of interest in activities	Write it down, and keep to a strict daily routine Baby steps makes it so much easier to get started with the tiny first step Create mutually agreed deadlines
Persistence & Perseverance	Tasks are almost never completed Inability to stick to a plan of action Cluttered and disorganized environment	Write down the plan and the steps to completion in the daily diary Develop a checklist that is interactive Start small

APPENDIX FIVE: BEHAVIOR

IMPAIRMENT	SYMPTOMS	TIPS
Control	Obsessive pondering of single ideas or thoughts Inappropriate comments Loss of inhibition Bad judgment Acts irrespective of consequences	Quietly move the discussion forward Clearly respond and explain inappropriate behavior or comments Discuss the consequences of possible behavior or comments Slow down the process
Self-Awareness	Underestimation of physical or cognitive impairments Lack of insight about the condition or consequences thereof.	Provide honest feedback Assume that the TBI survivor is not entirely aware of the parameters of his symptoms
Social	Misunderstand social boundaries Difficulty fitting in at social events Inappropriate reactions and comments Impulsive behavior	Establish signals to warn the person when they are overstepping Brief the person before participation in new social activities Provide constant feedback during the event to keep the person on track Carefully analyze and discuss inappropriate behavior afterward

APPENDIX SIX: EMOTION

IMPAIRMENT	SYMPTOMS	TIPS
Lack of control	Reduced ability to absorb frustration Inappropriate expression of emotion Mood swings	Remain calm at all times Do not react to surprising or unexpected behavior or reactions Help the person to calm down or become cognizant of their emotions Remember that this is the result of the injuries to the brain Give gentle and quiet feedback Allow the person the opportunity to talk and express their emotions and feelings

APPENDIX SEVEN: COMMUNICATION

IMPAIRMENT	SYMPTOMS	TIPS
Starting a conversation	Lack of response to a conversation Does not answer questions Prolonged and inappropriate pauses	Prompt the person and attempt to pull them into the conversation Be patient and give them enough time Do not become inattentive
Participating in conversation	Does not understand what people are saying to them Cannot concentrate long enough to follow the discussion Never stops talking Cannot fathom changes in the topic of conversation Has difficulty to keep to the topic Slurred speech, rapid speech or inaudible or too loud speech	Be concise Repeat what is being said. Attempt to keep eye contact Keep pulling the person back by getting their attention Interrupt and ask for an opportunity to respond or participate Clarify when new topics are taken on Ask the person to repeat until you can make out what he is saying Indicate if she is too loud or too rapid or too soft-spoken using cues and signals
Body Language	Oblivious to body language cues Invades people's personal space Inappropriate physical contact Disparities between body language and conversation Disconnected between expression and the content of the communication Disruptive movements while talking Lack of eye contact Inappropriate looking at or staring at others	Request the person give you a bit of personal space Express and explain to the person if inappropriate physical contact happens Ask the person if they are able to stop the disruptive movements they are making Ask the person if their expressions do not match their tone or conversational content, i.e., laughing at some suffering while expressing sadness, nevertheless. Indicate to the person that their staring or gaze is inappropriate or ask them to make eye contact if appropriate

Conclusion

Yes, it is a large topic, and no book can treat it with enough thoroughness and detail to include everything a reader might want to know or everything a patient might experience and require information about. In this work, I attempted to create a balance between practical advice and factual information to create a book that can both inform and educate without getting lost in unnecessary complexities or unsorted details.

What is important, is that this book has to be read as a statement of hope and as a declaration of faith - that no matter how bad things might appear at the beginning of the long road to recovery, faith and persistence, perseverance and hope will carry you and your loved ones to a better place, to a city of peace.

My journey was long, and sometimes I suffocated for lack of clarity and vision. I hope my readers will benefit from this work and will be able to pass the time on their own journeys with a bit more certainty, a bit more faith and a bit more belief for the efforts of those who came before them and those who came before me. Life is a journey. Enjoy the ride!

Finally, if you found this book useful in any way, a review on Amazon is always appreciated!

About the Authors

Leon Edward

It was 35 years ago that a bullet instantly switched off the "lights" for Leon Edward. When he "woke up" from the coma after his traumatic brain injury, he suffered from hemiparesis (partial paralysis) and the road to recovery stretched out before him. It was a long road indeed.

Leon had the support of an incredible medical team who nursed him along. Leon counts his blessing today. His physical and cognitive recovery was nothing short of miraculous, and despite all the adversity, Leon overcame.

First, he graduated as a Mechanical Engineer. As if this was not enough of an accomplishment, he was successful in business continuing personal improvement for the next 25 years.

For Leon the past 35 years since the TBI left one lingering desire: the need to give something back, a way to provide something meaningful for the families and loved ones of patients who now, or in the future, will face the same painful disruption of their lives and the same long journey he had to undertake such a long time ago.

This book was written by one deeply caring brother for his brothers and sisters suffering the same or even a worse fate after surviving traumatic brain injuries – and with deep admiration and appreciation for their families and caretakers who will help to guide them along.

For Leon, it has become an ingrained part of his existence to help others enjoy life after suffering serious injuries, even if it only means that he can help others who are disabled or living alone with words of hope, encouragement of inspiration.

The journey is long, the journey is tough, but the road is built on hope and leads to happy endings.

Dr. Anum Khan

A doctor by profession and writer by passion, Dr. Khan is an advocate of healthy living and wellness, both at the hospital and outside. She enjoys a healthy lifestyle, and it permeates through her writing. She strongly believes that living a healthy life should come naturally and is absolutely possible for everyone with the right knowledge and attitude.

She graduated from her medical school in 2017 and is planning her residency in Internal Medicine. Along with her career, she picked up writing professionally and now takes the opportunity to educate readers about what she knows best: healthcare.

This book is an effort to help patients, families, and caretakers about Traumatic Brain Injury, and is aimed to be your best guide on the subject with an easy, stepwise and practical approach.

She hopes this read will be an enriching experience and will help everyone in some way.

Additional Books

from Leon Edward on Amazon
AuthorPage http://amazon.com/author/leonedward

HEMIPARESIS LIVING [Paperback and Kindle]:
AFTER A STROKE OR BRAIN INJURY and Hemiparesis Living Care, Rehab at Home Tips Exercises: Safety and Effects as One-Sided Muscle Weakness, Stroke Paralysis, ... Foot Drop, Spasticity with Patient Insights

BRAIN INJURY PREVENTION AND SAFETY TIPS:
[Paperback and Kindle]: Reducing the Risk of Concussions and Traumatic Brain Injury in Sports and Activities!

UNDERSTANDING SPASTICITY
Living with Spasticity and Emotional Consequences, Safety and Care: Know the Effects on Life, Realistic Goals, Treatment Options, Exercises, Tips, Long Term Outlook

SPASTICITY STRETCHING EXERCISES: Stretch in your home easily even alone
Compilation of stretching exercises for spasticity, many which can be done easily and without the use of a partner at home. This guide of techniques to decrease spasticity was prepared by working along with an occupational therapist, using these

techniques for spasticity, drastic improvement in relief would increase movement was seen.

A GUIDE TO OVERCOMING LONELINESS AND HOPELESSNESS:

Positive Tips Techniques Advice How to Help People All Ages Find Happiness and Hope in Times of Trouble

HOW TO GUIDE MANAGE STRESS RELAX DON'T WORRY:

TIPS TECHNIQUES and CHECKLISTS for NATURAL Stress Management in MINUTES and ' How to END ANXIETY '... RELAX and get BETTER SLEEP:

Follow Leon Edward on Amazon and review books at author page Books: AuthorPage or http://amazon.com/author/leonedward

ENDNOTES

i   Original quote ascribed to Mark Twain: "Reports of my death are greatly exaggerated."

ii Stuss, D. T., Binns, M. A., Carruth, F. G., Levine, B., Brandys, C. E., Moulton, R. J., Schwartz, M. L. (1999). The acute period of recovery from traumatic brain injury: posttraumatic amnesia or posttraumatic confusional state? Journal of Neurosurgery, 90(4), 635–643. doi:10.3171/jns.1999.90.4.0635

iii The GAIN guideline "Guideline on Regional Immediate Discharge Documentation for Patients being discharged from Secondary into Primary Care."

iv An **anticholinergic** agent blocks the neurotransmitter acetylcholine in the central and the peripheral nervous system that inhibit parasympathetic nerve impulses.

v   McKee Celia A., Lukens John R. "Emerging Roles for the Immune System in Traumatic Brain Injury" Frontiers in Immunology, 7, 556 **AND** A. Houlden, M. Goldrick, D, et. al. Brain injury induces specific changes in the caecal microbiota of mice via altered autonomic activity and mucoprotein production. Brain, Behavior, and Immunity. 2016, 57, 10-20.

vi McMillan TM, Teasdale GM, Stewart E. Disability in young people and adults after head injury: 12-14 year follow-up of a prospective cohort. J Neurol Neurosurg Psychiatry. 2012; 83:1086–91.

vii Ulfarsson, T., "Predictors of long-term outcome after severe traumatic brain injury" Department of Clinical Neuroscience and Rehabilitation. Institute of Neuroscience and Physiology, Sahlgrenska Academy at University of Gothenburg, 2013

viii The World Federation of Occupational Therapy definition.

ix American Guide to Occupational Therapy Practice

x   Stocchetti and Zanier Critical Care (2016) 20:148 DOI 10.1186/s13054-016-1318-1

xi American Psychiatric Association. Diagnostic and Statistical Manual of Mental Disorders, (DSM V). 5th ed. Washington, DC: American Psychiatric Association; 2013

Made in the USA
Las Vegas, NV
29 December 2020